TABLE OF CONTENTS

"SAFE AND SIMPLE PROCEDURE"

Vasectomy is a "safe and simple procedure" according to many in the medical profession. While the simple part might be accurate, the safe part is definitely not. The cruelest cut of all frequently produces lifelong pain, often worsened by sexual activity, arising months or years after the procedure. Too ashamed to speak up many men suffer in silence unless the pain is severe. For those seeking treatment the options are confusing, expensive, not readily available, and in a worse case scenario involve removing a testicle. With vasectomy labeled as a "safe and simple procedure" by the medical community, men and their spouses are being grossly misled.

Post-Vasectomy Pain Syndrome (PVPS) truly represents the tip of the proverbial iceberg, and the concern of physicians and researchers as to why this supposedly rare complication occurs is incredibly misdirected, because the theoretical and practical foundation supporting vasectomy is hopelessly flawed. Take a pump and a balloon. As the balloon fills you reduce the pumping pressure and then stop. Now pump up another balloon and do not stop. A young child can predict what will happen—pressure will build and the balloon will burst.

In a similar fashion the testicles do not stop or greatly reduce sperm production after a vasectomy. Instead sperm production continues unabated as Sir Ashley Cooper noted way back in 1823 when he performed vasectomies upon dogs. Pressure builds leading to "blow-outs" or slow leakage of sperm, both capable of triggering inflammatory reactions and severe pain. What is truly amazing is that most vasectomized men do not experience chronic pain, a real testi-

1

mony to the compensatory and healing powers of the body and not to the success of the procedure. For those of you who are thinking that the problem shows up soon after a vasectomy and would have shown up by now if you have already been vasectomized, think again—chronic pain can arise at any time, commonly 5 to 7 years and even ten or more years after the procedure.

Physicians and contraception counselors usually downplay the pain aspect of vasectomy. Often there is no warning about ongoing pain, or the risk is stated to be very low and the problem treatable surgically. That such advice is given is amazing considering that research studies have quoted figures as high as 18.7%, 27.2%, 33% and even up to 54% for Post-Vasectomy Pain Syndrome! Furthermore, when it comes to resolving a problem that should never have arisen in the first place, almost never is it mentioned that multiple operations might be required for even a modest reduction in symptoms.

Surgical reversal of a vasectomy is commonly hailed as the corrective treatment of choice. Rarely is it indicated that this procedure quite often fails to resolve the pain and might only work for a limited period of time, the latter a fact that even very few physicians are aware of. Nor is it mentioned that vasectomy reversals are generally not covered by insurance plans and are extremely costly due to the microsurgical skill required, equipment, and length of the procedure. Even more astonishing is the spread of vasectomy to third world countries promoted as a "safe and simple" form of birth control. In these settings the surgical skill and equipment for reversal operations are essentially nonexistent, and very few could afford the procedure even assuming that surgeons and equipment were available. To promote this procedure to men in general is seriously misguided, but to advocate it for men who cannot access any potentially effective treatment for PVPS is nothing short of horrendous.

The contraceptive success of vasectomy is often cited as such a plus that it makes the risk worthwhile. True if there were only short-term surgical complications such as wound infections. Not so if a procedure is fundamentally flawed theoretically and practically, and in such a way that chronic discomfort and pain frequently occur. The thinking of physicians and contraception counselors must break away from the current fixation on vasectomy as a "safe and simple procedure" to vasectomy as a dangerous and even cruel procedure. If you are considering having a vasectomy or have already been vasectomized, know someone in either situation, provide contraception counseling, or perform vasectomies and/or corrective surgery, read on to fully understand and appreciate why vasectomy might well be the cruelest cut of all.

NATURE LEFT ALONE

Anatomy and physiology frighten away many people, physicians included. Fortunately, the science associated with vasectomy is quite straightforward at a basic level and many commonly held misconceptions about male anatomy are quickly revealed for what they are, to be replaced by a solid grasp of what is actually occurring within and beyond the scrotum.

TESTICLES:

Although a symbol of virility and undeniably crucial to being a man, the internal workings seem like a mystery to most. Given the obvious importance of reproduction in the context of evolution, it is not surprising that nature has built redundancy into the system by providing two testicles. One testicle can easily take care of the job at hand. Each of these little wonders of nature is divided into about 250 compartments each containing 1-4 small tubes, referred to as seminiferous tubules, where sperm is produced. From start to finish the process takes about 70 days or over 2 months—a baby only takes a little more than 6 months longer. Sertoli cells within each tubule stimulate the growth of sperm and provide nourishment as they develop. Another type-Leydig cells-situated between the tubules produce male hormones, such as testosterone, responsible for the growth and maintenance of secondary sexual features including facial hair and deep voice.

The adult testicle produces about 4.25 million sperm per gram and the average testicle weighs 16.9 grams. Close to 7,000,000,000 sperm are produced by each testicle!

4

However, only about 50% to 60% eventually enter into the ejaculate. The volume of each ejaculation is approximately 3 milliliters, the contribution of the testicles with sperm and secretions is only 5-10% of the total ejaculate volume. Within the ejaculate there is about 100 million sperm per milliliter, unquestionably a lot of sperm. It appears that nature wanted to make sure that in case a few were not functioning so well there will be some extra ones, as in several million additional contenders for the illustrious reproduction assignment.

EFFERENT DUCTS & EPIDIDYMIS:

Once their growth in the testicle is complete sperm are ready to fertilize the female egg. Wrong! Sperm taken from the testis are inactive and unable to fertilize an egg without special assistance. At the upper pole (top) of the testicle sperm pass into numerous efferent, meaning out, ducts feeding into the top section (head) of the epididymis. The epididymis, now there is a word, is a highly coiled organ that extends from the upper pole of each testicle to the bottom (lower pole) on one side. If a cut is made into the epididymis several tubules are noted due to the coiling, but there is only one tube about 20 ft in length. The middle portion is the body and the lower portion of the epididymis, referred to as the tail, bends at the ductus deferens where it connects with the vas deferens, the latter organ cut when a vasectomy is performed.

Sperm are transformed into fully functioning entities within the efferent ducts and epididymis elevating these organs from the simple conduits once thought to be to a crucial reproductive structure. Of particular significance, sperm become motile during their passage through the epididymis. Beyond the illustrious role of maturing sperm, the efferent ducts and epididymis reabsorb the 40% to 50% or so of sperm that are not functional or have abnormalities.

In addition, the epididymis and possibly the efferent ducts add secretions. Both structures move sperm from the testicle by contraction of so-called smooth muscles within the ducts and coils, and also by the sweeping action of small hair-like structures called cilia. If you are feeling overwhelmed by these odd words take pride that by the end you might almost have learned another language. It has been said that the average medical student learns the equivalent of 4 or so languages in terms of the number of words that are required to get by. Now back to more anatomy.

The fundamental shift in perceived function of the efferent ducts and epididymis by medical researchers and physicians demonstrates how nature is more complex than we often like to think, and how all organs do have a significant function. Medical researchers not infrequently cite structures, such as the epididymis and appendix, as having no or minimal functions when they do not yet understand what the true function is.

VAS DEFERENS:

More commonly referred to as the vas, this very unique tube runs continuous from the tail of the epididymis (that word again), eventually to connect with the urethra, the tube carrying urine and the products of ejaculation out of the body. Valves within the reproductive structures prevent backflow of urine or other secretions. The vas is the most unique tube within the human body because it is the only tubular organ, male or female, where the diameter of the lumen (space inside) is less than the thickness of the wall. The lumen is an incredibly small 0.5 millimeters with a maximum diameter of about 1.5 millimeters, about the width of a printed letter. This small lumen and thick wall design emphasizes the function of the vas—to propel sperm and associated secretions out of the body. It also suggests that any scarring in the thick wall could easily block the lumen.

The relatively thick wall of the vas consists of an outer covering (the adventitia), a 3 layer muscle section, and the inner part (the mucosa). The 3-layer muscle is comprised of inner and outer layers running lengthwise and a middle circular layer, an arrangement providing a great deal of propulsive strength. A complex plexus of nerves running parallel to and surrounding the vas stimulates the muscle contractions. The combined propulsive actions of the efferent ducts, epididymis, and vas leave little doubt that the system is entirely designed by nature to get mature and viable sperm out as efficiently as possible, a state of affairs that should prompt any informed and logical person to think twice, or ten times for that matter, about doing anything to interrupt the flow.

SEMINAL VESICLES & PROSTATE:

Joining the vas to form an ejaculatory duct is a seminal vesicle, a soft 6 centimeter structure. The seminal vesicles contribute about 60% of the fluid comprising the ejaculate. Further along the system is the prostate, a glandular organ surrounding the start of the urethra. The prostate's contribution to the ejaculate volume is approximately 30% and consists of a milky component. If the ejaculate ever becomes watery and not at all cloudy, consider the possibility of blockage of the prostate due to inflammation or infection. Clearly, secretions from the seminal vesicles and prostate comprise the bulk of the ejaculate. Hence, the reduction in ejaculate volume after vasectomy is rarely noticeable to the naked eye. Any significant reduction should alert a clinician to the possibility of inflammation or infection of the prostate or seminal vesicles, resulting in reduced secretions from one or both of these structures.

TAMPERING WITH NATURE

In simple terms the vas is cut during a vasectomy—ectomy is a suffix used to denote removal of any anatomical structure. Closed-ended and open-ended refer to the two basic types of vasectomy, with the former being much more commonly performed worldwide. Although there are several different techniques, both types of vasectomy typically involve removal of 10-15 millimeters of each vas deferens and management of the exposed ends. This management can involve one or combinations of sewing (ligature) often first folding a segment of the vas over itself, cautery (burning), clipping, or placing fibrous tissue covering the vas over the open end and sewing it off (fascial interposition). By definition, open-ended vasectomies leave the testicular end of the vas open. The prostate end is sealed off usually by fascial interposition and sometimes cautery. The failure rate, defined as achieving pregnancy or the presence of motile sperm in the ejaculate following clearance of any residual sperm requiring up to about 15 ejaculations, is well below 1%.

From the minute, or even second, that a closed-ended vasectomy has been performed there is a huge increase in pressure within the testicle side of the vas that proves difficult for the system to cope with. In contrast, no pressure increase at all is found on the prostate side. At least two characteristics of the reproductive system set the stage for trouble. The first is that distressing evolutionary driven tendency for the testicle to just keep on producing sperm and secretions as if nothing at all happened. I guess we have got to try and reproduce no matter what. Even when a man is born without a vas on one or both sides-yes it does occur-the testicles act as if everything was fine with active sperm production. Another way of looking at it is that there is no feedback mechanism as there are in other tubular structures within the body. If the ureter-the tube connecting the kidney to the bladder-is severed the kidney on that side will eventually reduce and stop urine production. This relieves and extinguishes any pressure-induced damage to the kidney. I think some urologists must have been asleep for the lectures on hydrostatic pressure increases. As Sherman Silber mentions in his paper—Reversal of Vasectomy and the Treatment of Male Infertility—published in Urology Clinics of North America, 1981, "Most clinicians performing vasectomy have been totally ignorant of its pressure-mediated effects on the epididymis and testis."

The second characteristic that sets the stage for trouble is how the vas is the only tubular structure within the human body where the thickness of the wall is greater than the space inside. The strong smooth muscles in the wall keep pushing sperm and secretions down to the site of the obstruction. In addition, the thick wall enables sperm to enter it in significant numbers setting the stage for an inflammatory reaction. Starting with the vas and working back to the testicle let us see what changes result from the cruelest cut of all.

VAS DEFERENS:

Stanwood Schmidt and Erich Brueschke way back in 1976 in their study—Anatomical Sizes Of The Human Vas Deferens After Vasectomy—published in Fertility And Sterility, looked at how the vas dilates following a vasectomy. To investigate this they measured the vas in 22 men who were undergoing vasectomy reversal, a procedure that reconnects the severed vas. The men in their study were vasectomized 1 to 19 years before. Sizing of the lumen was based on the largest gauge that could be introduced, a nice way of saying inserted. I do hope these men were under general anesthesia.

The average diameter of the lumen on the testicle side was 1.73 millimeters with a standard deviation (variance around the average) of .29 mm. On the prostate side the mean diameter was 1.03 mm with a standard deviation of .20 mm. Hence, the average increase in luminal diameter of the testicular side after vasectomy was 0.7 mm or about 70%! Interestingly, the external size of the vas was the same for both sides, clearly indicating that the dilation of the testicular side involves a thinning of the wall and not an increase in external diameter. When there is no dilation it is either the case that the testis is not producing sperm or that there is an obstruction further from the site of the vasectomy, such as the epididymis.

Barry Shandling and Joseph Janik—The Vulnerability Of The Vas Deferens, Journal of Pediatric Surgery, 1981—conducted experiments with rats, whereby they briefly clamped the vas different ways and six weeks later examined each vas. Even with mild techniques, inflammatory reactions were observed both in the lumen and in the wall of the vas. The inflammatory reactions were so-called, sterile, because there was no infection.

Given that simply clamping the vas briefly, at least in rats, can produce an inflammatory reaction, it would seem almost certain that a vasectomy could result in this problem. Assuming that sperm does make it to the vas it is inevitably going to accumulate when a closed-ended vasectomy has been completed. Accumulated sperm often extravasates, meaning that it passes out of the lumen into the wall. Imagine a flexible tube carrying water that is blocked at the end. Pressure needs to be released at some point to limit damage to the pumping system, and it does so by breaking through the inner wall of the water hose and spreading between the inner and outer layers dissecting them apart. In plumbing the hose is more likely to split open spilling water all over. Biology appears to have devised a better solution by allowing fluids to spread between layers thereby forestalling or preventing a complete rupture.

When sperm extravasates a so-called sperm granuloma forms, the two main sites being the section of the vas that has been blocked (vasectomy site) and the epididymis. Stuart McDonald—Cellular Responses To Vasectomy— published in International Review of Cytology (2000) describes sperm granulomas as rounded or irregular in shape, 1 millimeter to 1 centimeter or more, with a central mass of degenerating sperm surrounded by tissue containing blood vessels and immune system cells. Interestingly, they resemble the granulomas of tuberculosis possibly because sperm contain fatty acids similar to those released by tubercle bacteria leading to a similar type of immune system response.

Sherman Silber in performing over a thousand vasectomy reversal operations with the aid of an operating microscope, always observed some degree of vas lumen dilatation, as reported in Reversal of Vasectomy and the Treatment of Male Infertility. He discovered that the presence of a sperm granuloma at the vasectomy site virtually guaranteed good quality sperm in the vas fluid demonstrating the pressure and consequent damage reducing effects of sperm granulomas. In an earlier article—Vasectomy And Vasectomy Reversal (Fertility And Sterility,1978) Sherman Silber noted that when a sperm granuloma is only found on one side, sperm quality is good on that side, but worse on the side lacking a sperm granuloma. He comments that a sperm granuloma at the vasectomy site represents a safety release valve helping to alleviate the high buildup of pressure. Hence, sperm granulomas should not be viewed as complications of a closed-ended vasectomy.

Stanwood Schmidt, the same as in Schmidt and Brueschke, in his study—Spermatic Granuloma: An Often Painful Lesion, Fertility And Sterility 1979—examined over

100 sperm granulomas and described them as asymptomatic (no pain) or symptomatic (painful), even agonizingly so at times. According to Schmidt asymptomatic granulomas result from either minor, non-progressive leakage of sperm or to a long existing lesion. In either case there is a stabilizing layer of epithelial cells (lining cells) and all inflammation resolves. Symptomatic granulomas, in contrast, always have a wall of inflammatory cells. These granulomas are often cystic; a cyst is an abnormal sac containing gas, liquid, or some semisolid material, with a membranous lining. Contents of granuloma cysts consist of decapitated sperm (no mercy here), red blood cells, and immune system cells designed to clear cellular debris. To wall off the inflammation fibrous tissue forms around the granuloma, and of particular importance to PVPS—nerves can be entrapped in this fibrous tissue. It does not take a pain specialist to figure out what might occur.

The introduction of sperm into the wall of the vas, epididymis, or efferent ducts sets off an inflammatory reaction because the body does not recognize sperm as belonging to itself! While inside the tubules where sperm grow, mature and pass out of the penis, sperm are actually outside the body proper, much as food is inside your colon. Sperm are first produced at puberty by which time the immune system has recognized all body components. The newly formed sperm are alien to the body, and a blood-testes barrier prevents sperm from being detected by the immune system.

Once sperm extravasate from the lumen the immune system detects them and initiates a search and destroy operation of sorts. Beyond the specialized cells that are recruited to take out the sperm (there are no prisoners as far as the immune system is concerned) antibodies frequently form to tag the sperm for destruction. Sounds somewhat like the US armed forces but probably much more effective. These antibodies are known as antisperm antibodies and are the focus of concerns that vasectomy might have negative effects on other organs, such as the heart and prostate by setting up a system wide autoimmune attack. This remains a highly controversial subject to be dealt with in a later chapter.

If all these vasectomy induced changes to the vas seem like enough fun wait because there is more. Remember all that smooth muscle in the walls of the efferent ducts, epididymis, and vas moving sperm and testicular secretions along. In a very interesting couple of studies Shafik—Electrovasogram In Normal And Vasectomized Men And Patients With Obstructive Azoospermia And Absent Vas Deferens, Archives Of Andrology, 1996—examined the electrical activity of the vas. In the first study it was shown that the vas has two forms of electrical activity—slow waves or pacesetter potentials (PPs) and action potentials (APs), the latter associated with increased pressure within the vas indicative of movement. This study was conducted using dogs as subjects.

The second study by Shafik sought to compare healthy subjects as pertains to reproductive functioning, men with obstruction, and men who had reversal surgery. Electrodes placed on the scrotum measured electrical activity of the vas. The electrovasogram (yes, another one of those words) in healthy subjects showed PPs that were solid and consistent on all test days. The frequency, amplitude, velocity of conduction, and time between cycles were stable. APs representing fast spike activity followed some but not all PPs. Turning to vasectomized subjects the PPs on the testicular side of the vas were diminished in terms of frequency and amplitude compared to normal subjects. They also had an irregular rhythm and their frequency and amplitude were inconsistent in each individual on all test days. In short, the PPs showed an abnormal rhythm—vasoarrhythmia. In some subjects silent periods were recorded where there was no activity at all. There were no APs at all in any of the subjects.

Pressure level and electrical activity in the vas of men undergoing reversal surgery also proved very revealing. The pressure level on the prostate side was normal, but the pressure level on the testicular side displayed a significant pressure increase reflecting the problem of ongoing sperm production relative to inadequate compensatory mechanisms. Electrovasograms showed an absence of PPs and APs in the prostate end and vasoarrythmias in the testicular end. 1 to 6 years after reversal surgery the electrovasogram yielded different patterns. Some had normal patterns, some had regular rhythms but diminished frequency and amplitude, and some showed vasoarrythmias. Quite amazing, although largely to be expected, the men with normal electrical activity in the vas were more likely to impregnate their wives. Those who demonstrated a regular but diminished rhythm were also likely to achieve pregnancy. No pregnancies occurred when the vasoarrythymia persisted after reversal. These results clearly demonstrate the importance of electrical activity within the vas for the purpose of effectively propelling sperm along, and how much damage vasectomies can inflict on the electrical activity of the vas.

EFFERENT DUCTS & EPIDIDYMIS:

Impairment of vas functioning brings impairment in other organs on the testicular side largely due to pressure buildup and accumulation of sperm. Way back in 1976 Dev Pardanani, Nivrutti Patil, and Hindurao Pawar in their study— Some Gross Observations Of The Epididymis Following Vasectomy: A Clinical Study, published in Fertility And Sterility—examined 220 epididymides from 114 vasectomized men during reversal surgery. In 150 (68%) swelling, distension, and fullness was observed. Of these 150 epididymides 44 (29%) showed ducts filled with whitish material.

Examination under the microscope revealed sperm in various stages of breakdown. In 3 instances there were actual cysts representing cystic sperm granulomas. A further 25 (16.6%) had tense and cyst-like areas in the upper section (head).

Pardanani, Patil, and Pawar concluded that the changes observed were indicative of an imbalance between the rates of sperm and testicular fluid production on the one hand and their reabsorption in the efferent ducts and epididymis on the other hand. Furthermore, the changes observed likely impaired sperm maturation—recall that the epididymis plays a key role in the growth of sperm and in the absence of this structure sperm are not able to fertilize eggs. Edward Shapiro and Sherman Silber—Open-Ended Vasectomy, Sperm Granuloma, And Postvasectomy Orchalgia,1979, in Fertility And Sterility—reported that in more than 800 vas reversal surgery patients, with only some reversals due to pain, they have always observed some degree of epididymal enlargement and congestion. Getting right to the point they wrote—"Indeed after one explores these post-vasectomy patients microsurgically, it becomes difficult to understand why the vast majority of such patients have no pain or discomfort." Aside from the, vast majority part, the comment is very insightful.

Moving ahead to the eighties Jarvis and Dubbins—Changes In The Epididymis After Vasectomy: Sonographic Findings, American Journal Of Roenten., 1989—applied ultrasound to examine 31 men before and after vasectomy. They discovered that after vasectomy the epididimydes enlarged and cysts formed. Applying a technique by which the epididymis is removed to control pain, Stuart Selowitz and Alan Schned were able to study these organs carefully, their classic research paper—A Late Post-Vasectomy Syndrome—published in The Journal Of Urology, 1985. Removal of the epididymis allowed the symptoms reported by individual men to be linked with detailed findings. The pain experienced by their subjects was constant and often disabling. It typically worsened with sexual activity, and in some cases radiated to other spermatic cord structures.

In the case of A.R. a 1 cm mass would form at the lower end of the epididymis and on the following day he would suffer a worsening of pain. Then the swelling and pain would diminish. Like with many of the other men (18 total in this study) the epididymis was nodular (full of small and hard ball-like structures). There were numerous sperm granulomas, dilated tubules so large that they could almost be seen clearly without the aid of a microscope, inflammation, and extravasated sperm. No wonder A.R. experienced pain and that the pain disappeared after removal of the epididymis. In another case a dead mass of tissue was found in the epididymis leading the surgeons to remove both the epididymis and testicle.

Summarizing the results for all their patients in the study, Selikowitz and Schned indicated that the most common finding was dilated tubules, often massively so. Both dilated and nondilated tubules were frequently packed with sperm and histiocytes—inflammatory cells designed to remove cell debris. In several cases extravasated sperm was present, often producing sperm granulomas. Data from 20 epididymal specimens yielded the following results:

- Tubular dilation 17/20

- Packing of tubules (with sperm and inflammatory cells) 11/20

- Extravasation of sperm 9/20

- Sperm granulomas 7/20

Chen and Ball in their 1991 study, Epididymectomy For Post-Vasectomy Pain: Histological Review, 1991, published in the British Journal of Urology, conducted a similar study removing the epididymis on both sides in 10 patients and on one side in 5 patients suffering from PVPS, and then examining 24 of these. Epididymectomy was performed between 6 months and 20 years after vasectomy, with an average of 7 years. The onset of pain ranged from 1 month to 20 years after vasectomy, the average being 6 years. It is important to note that over half the patients had an onset beyond 6 years with one at 20 years! Regarding the pain itself, 14 patients experienced a constant dull ache in the scrotum and the remaining patient experienced constant severe pain. The pain was exacerbated during physical activity with 4 patients and during sexual intercourse with 3. At the time of surgery they dissected the epididymis from the neurovascular (nerves and blood vessels) bundle and removed the epididymis plus the section of the vas closest to it.

Detailed examination of the epididymides and efferent ducts revealed dilation of the ducts and fibrosis of the connective tissue supporting the ducts. All sections of the epididymis and efferent ductules were affected to a similar degree. There was also significant thickening of the muscle layer of the epididymal duct. Of tremendous significance for our understanding of PVPS, Chen and Ball noted nerves "densely encased" in fibrous tissue, with obvious distortion and twisting of the affected nerves in some cases! Nerves were more likely to be enveloped by fibrous tissue where the fibrosis was most extensive, mainly when this occurred in the tail of the epididymis. In one subject infiltration of immune system cells was detected around the nerves, implying an ongoing chronic inflammatory process affecting the nerves. They mention that under such conditions nerves are actually invaded by inflammatory cells. Their striking evidence of fibrosis around nerves, referred to as perineural fibrosis, and related processes provides abundant reason for the pain experienced by those suffering from Post-Vasectomy Pain Syndrome.

Neither Selikowitz and Schned or Chen and Ball detected any sign of infection. This is an extremely important point because it is common for physicians to assume that there is an infection of the epididymis and prescribe antibiotics. Many PVPS patients have been prescribed several antibiotics often to be taken over long periods of time. This practice for the most part constitutes a waste of time, not to mention a waste of financial resources, because the pain has nothing to do with infection. The exception is when there has been an infection in the prostate or perhaps some other organ in the region prior to vasectomy. Prostate infections can be relatively pain free and persist for a long time. Vasectomy might potentially release the infection from the prostate side of the severed vas.

Following at least closed-ended vasectomy the build up in pressure encourages sperm granuloma formation either in the vas or epididymis to vent the system and prevent more severe damage. Sherman Silber (1981) believes that it is simply a question of which of these two sites the sperm granuloma will appear at. Furthermore, multiple sperm granulomas can form in the epididymis. Stuart MacDonald (2000) demonstrated the presence of multiple epididymal granulomas indicating abundant sperm leakage. Apparently, these granulomas can drain sperm for a while and then seal off, possibly re-opening later as part of an ongoing and dynamic process to vent pressure.

Increased hydrostatic pressure produces a thinning of the epithelial (inner) lining of the tubule, increasing the likelihood of breaks and sperm extravasation at that location. Thinning of the epididymal epithelial layer might also impair the maturation of sperm. Karine Doiron and colleagues— Effect of Vasectomy on Gene Expression in the Epididymis of Cynomolgus Monkey—published in Biology Of Reproduction (2002) discovered that pressure induced thinning of the epithelium of the epididymis diminishes the formation of proteins necessary for sperm to become motile, a prerequisite for successful unaided fertilization of the egg. These researchers conclude that the fate of the epididymis after vasectomy depends on the elasticity of the epididymal tubules, amount of spermatozoa produced, and the reabsorption capacity of the epididymis.

Epididymal sperm granulomas are indeed common following vasectomy. Shapiro and Silber (1979) reported sperm granuloma formation in the epididymis on one side in 10% of men who have had their vasectomy less than 10 years ago and on both sides in 50% of men who had their vasectomy greater than 10 years ago. Recalling how the testicles continue to produce sperm and associated fluids as if nothing happened, and how smooth muscles in the efferent ducts, epididymis, and vas attempt to propel these products out, it is understandable why Shapiro and Silber way back in 1979 proposed that increased hydrostatic pressure following vasectomy results in dilation and distension of the epididymis, and is responsible for epididymal blow-outs and subsequent sperm granuloma formation. Such granulomas have been referred to as secondary; primary granulomas arise from the less dramatic process of sperm leakage (mini blow-outs of sorts) at the vasectomy site in the vas or the epididymis, combined with the reaction of the immune system to the foreign sperm. Nature is truly amazing and sometimes only reveals how much so when it is tampered with.

Research pertaining to the efferent duct—the organ connecting the testicle to the epididymis—is extremely limited. Apparently, this neglected organ has fallen into a research abyss between more esteemed neighbors. Considering that in many ways it functions like the epididymis, several of the same vasectomy-related problems likely plague it. Sherman Silber (1978) reported that obstruction of the head of the epididymis (where it connects with the efferent ducts) blocks outflow of sperm and secretions, the impact on the efferent ducts consisting of fragmentation of the epithelial lining cells and degenerating sperm.

In their 2003 review article—Testicular Pain Follow-ing Vasectomy: A Review Of Postvasectomy Pain Syn-drome, published in the Journal of Andrology—Cory Christiansen and Jay Sandlow propose that the efferent ducts and epididymis (apparently the efferent ducts cannot have any fame on their own) absorb dead and degrading sperm through epithelial cells lining the walls. With a vasectomy the capacity of these cells to absorb sperm is entirely over-whelmed leading to cell gobbling macrophages, much like the now ancient Pac man, being recruited from the blood stream to assist with the digestion and clearance of the nonfunctioning sperm. In addition, the epithelial cells that normally absorb sperm weaken at their junctions allowing some sperm to extravasate and initiate a more extensive inflammatory reaction. Following vasectomy the cells that move sperm die and wall thickness increases. The diameter of the ducts is also altered increasing 2 to 4 times.

Chen and Ball (1991) detected pronounced dilation of the efferent ducts and interstitial fibrosis. There were so-called "brown patches" in 10 of the 24 epididymides and efferent ducts examined. These "brown patches" marked discolored areas of dilated ductules containing impacted sperm and cellular debris, with fibrosis and inflammatory cells in the spaces between the tubules. Evidently neither the efferent ducts or the epididymis get off lightly with a vasectomy.

TESTICLES:

Now we come to the start of the line in terms of fertility and the end of the line in terms of backpressure forces arising from a vasectomy. Clearly the vas and epididymis suffer greatly from a vasectomy even if there is no pain. Could it be that the testicles are spared. Unfortunately not, according to Jonathan Jarrow and fellow researchers in their 1985 paper—Quantitative Pathologic Changes In The Human

Testes After Vasectomy—published in the New England Journal of Medicine. They compared testicular samples taken from 31 men seeking vasectomy reversal for the purpose of restoring fertility to testicular samples taken from 21 men who had not been vasectomized. The comparison focused on the following parameters:

- Thickness of the walls of the seminiferous tubules (where sperm mature and are later conducted to the efferent ducts).

- Average cross-sectional area within the seminiferous tubules.

- Number of Sertoli cells—support the maturing sperm.

- Number of mature sperm.

- Fibrosis (hardening) of the space between the tubules.

Right across the board they found the following clear evidence of damage to the vasectomized testicles:

- Samples from vasectomized men showed a 100% increase in the thickness of the seminiferous tubular walls, compared to the samples from normal testicles.

- A 50% increase in the average cross-sectional area within the seminiferous tubules was observed in the vasectomized samples.

- Number of Sertoli cells was significantly reduced in the vasectomized samples relative to the healthy ones.

- Number of mature sperm was significantly reduced in the vasectomized samples.

- No fibrosis was observed in the normal testicles but seen in 23% of the samples from vasectomized men.

Increases in both wall thickness and average cross sectional area within seminiferous tubules are directly related to a buildup of pressure and adjustment to this insult. Reduced number of Sertoli cells almost certainly results from vasectomy-initiated damage, greatly limiting the support that can be given to maturing sperm. Consequently, there are fewer mature sperm. Fibrosis of the space between the tubules is not as easy to understand but does have a very significant impact—Jarrow and fellow researchers found that none of the men who achieved pregnancy after the reversal surgery showed fibrosis, whereas over 50% of the men who did not achieve fertility demonstrated fibrosis! Furthermore, none of the men with fibrosis achieved fertility

Supporting the findings by Jonathan Yarrow is the work by Japanese researchers Koji Shiraishi, Hiroshi Takibara and Katsusuke Naito—Influence Of Interstitial Fibrosis On Spermatogenesis After Vasectomy And Vasovasotomy—published in Contraception 2002. These researchers obtained testicular biopsies from 21 men who were being operated on to reverse their vasectomy. Fibrosis was observed around the tubules producing sperm (peritubular fibrosis) and also in the interstitial tissue including around blood vessels (perivascular fibrosis).

Shiraishi's team also found the percent of fibrosis to be a major factor in achieving pregnancy—the higher the percent of fibrosis the lower the pregnancy rate. They speculate that fibrotic tissue may prevent the compliance of the seminiferous tubules thereby reducing sperm production. Koji Shiraishi in another article—Vasectomy Impairs

Spermatogenesis Through Germ Cell Apoptosis Mediated By The p53-Bax Pathway In Rats—published in the Journal Of Urology in 2001, discovered that increased hydrostatic pressure impairs sperm maturation via apoptosis which, as opposed to necrosis, is an active process guiding cell development and delay. Increased pressure in the testicles seems to increase p53 tumor suppressor, thereby suppressing the maturation of sperm. They speculate based on other research that apoptosis only occurs when there is a pressure increase and that the presence of a sperm granuloma blocks this affect by venting pressure.

An alternative explanation for the testicular changes observed after vasectomy is the initiation of inflammatory autoimmune reactions. Investigating this possibility Jonathan Yarrow's group examined the walls of the seminiferous tubules for signs of inflammation but could not detect any. They note that other researchers have failed to find antisperm antibodies in these walls following vasectomy. Adding further evidence against the inflammation possibility, Koji Shiraishi's team discovered that the level of antisperm antibodies did not have any impact on the testicular changes observed.

Conditions such as congenital absence of the vas deferens (born without the vas) where inflammation is not a concern, reveal similar damage of the seminiferous tubules as sperm continues to be produced with no where to go. That the damage appears to be less than with an abrupt blockage later in life, as with vasectomy, suggests that the testicles might have some way of adapting when the problem arises early in life. Manuel Nistal and fellow researchers— Testicular Biopsy In Patients With Obstructive Azoospermia—published in the American Journal of Surgical Pathology (1999), also found that with all blockages including vasectomy, there tended to be fewer mature sperm indicating that while sperm numbers might not be affected the quality of sperm is. Providing an interesting comparison between the impact of vasectomy on testicular functioning to a complete blockage of ureter outflow for kidney functioning, Yarrow points out that the walls of the kidney can thicken 2 to 3 times to compensate for the increase in hydrostatic pressure and the kidney can greatly reduce outflow over time thereby reducing the pressure experienced within the system.

The impact of backpressure on the testicle appears to mainly affect the region by the efferent ducts and is less pronounced elsewhere according to Sherman Silber (1978). Stewart MacDonald (2000) reports that a key factor is the presence of sperm granulomas in the head of the epididymis, the section where the efferent ducts connect. Apparently granulomas of the epididymal head cannot accommodate the sperm and fluid produced by the testes, perhaps because they compress this narrow segment linking the efferent ducts to the body of the epididymis. Failure to vent pressure leads to backpressure within the testicle and degeneration of the epithelial lining of the seminiferous tubules of the testes near to the efferent ducts. In rats with sperm granulomas in this region the testicles can swell to twice their normal size. Human testes have a tougher covering around the testicles so they do not swell but damage can certainly transpire. Stuart MacDonald emphasizes that the belief held by many re-searchers and clinicians that vasectomy has no effect on the testis is simply not true.

In contrast to the obvious damage to the sperm pro-ducing Sertoli cells, at least in the absence of sperm granu-lomas, there does not appear to be any impact on Leydig cells and the production or release of male hormones. These cells are situated between the seminiferous tubules containing Sertoli cells and developing sperm. Whyte and colleagues—The Vasectomized Testis—published in International Surgery (2000) performed vasectomies on rats and discov-ered that although there was a marked increase in collagen fibers (fibrosis) of the space between the tubules the Leydig cells were unaffected. Of course this result was found for rats and there are many differences between various species and even different specific strains of a given type of animal, but no alteration in Leydig cell appearance or testosterone production has been reliably observed in humans. Theoretically, however, if there was enough damage due to fibrosis, excretion of testosterone from the testes might be impaired.

TIME SEQUENCE CHANGES FOLLOWING VASECTOMY:

In their informative and revealing article Christiansen and Sandlow review post-vasectomy changes distinguishing early, middle, and late, providing an important time sequence perspective on the aftereffects of vasectomy. They focus on changes associated with the more commonly practiced closed-ended vasectomy.

Early Post-Vasectomy Changes: When the vas is cut and blocked fluid pressure increases immediately and is transferred back to the source of the fluid-testes, efferent ducts, and epididymis. Initially, the diameter of the efferent ducts increases 2 to 4 times to counteract the increased pressure, and fluid absorption rises. The efferent ducts experience further changes in that the walls thicken and sperm moving cells with small hair like cilia disappear. Meanwhile sperm production continues unabated by the testicles clearly indicating that no feedback mechanism exists to reduce sperm production in response to outflow reduction or obstruction. Sperm produced are often not as mature likely due to a reduction in the number of Sertoli cells in the testicles. It has been suggested that these cells are very sensitive to pressure increases.

Intermediate Post-Vasectomy Changes: Christiansen and Sandlow indicate that the transition from early to intermediate post-vasectomy changes occurs when the fluid within the ejaculatory system overwhelms the ability of the efferent ducts and epididymis to accommodate the increase by dilating and reabsorbing. At this point macrophages are drawn in from the bloodstream to help digest the accumulating sperm. In rhesus monkeys this tends to occur around 3 months post-vasectomy when macrophages bloated with engulfed sperm drastically increase in numbers throughout the epididymis. Antisperm antibodies are likely to develop at this time as sperm leaks out of the inner space. In the case of rhesus monkeys almost all vasectomized males will have these antibodies within the epididymis, but antisperm antibodies only occur within the epididymis in 7% to 30% of men.

Late Post-Vasectomy Changes: Late phase changes are basically the result of compensatory responses to spare the testicle from serious damage arising from the sustained pressure increase. A key feature is the formation of sperm granulomas as sperm extravasates out of the inner space. Sperm granulomas also arise from so-called epididymal blow-outs—rupture of the walls of the epididymis due to unrelenting pressure. You might think that such a dramatic event is rare, yet one-sided blow-outs occur in 10% of patients within 10 years of vasectomy and blow-outs on both sides in 50% of patients greater than 10 years after vasectomy. Evidently, the problem is not so rare.

I believe it is painfully obvious to those who read the literature that the ejaculatory system does not get much of a break following vasectomy with what appears to be horrendous, but often fairly silent damage spreading throughout the system. With no feedback mechanism to reduce or shut down sperm production it continues with at most a very limited slowdown, and then only from damage to the seminiferous tubules and Sertoli cells of the testes. Overwhelmed by the fluid volume and pressure the efferent ducts, epididymis, and vas attempt to compensate but this eventually falters ushering in changes that in some vasectomized men result in the Post-Vasectomy Pain Syndrome.

THE INCIDENCE AND SYMPTOMS OF
POST-VASECTOMY PAIN SYNDROME

Pain can arise at any time following vasectomy from weeks to 10 or more years. For many it first manifests 5 to 7 years afterwards and is experienced as either sharp and severe, or more of a dull constant ache, and for the unlucky few there is both ongoing discomfort/pain and sharp stabbing pain with certain activities. Unfortunately, the testicles have a unique position outside the body because sperm require temperatures cooler than that of the body to mature. Regrettably, nature did not anticipate urologists and other physicians inflicting the damage they do. When things go wrong the exposed location of the testicles can turn simple activities such as sitting, exercising, sex, and even wearing coarse pants like jeans into a living nightmare.

Adding insult to injury many men who suffer from PVPS, particularly if the vasectomy was performed months or years prior, are misdiagnosed when they visit their family physician and prescribed antibiotics. When one or more courses of antibiotics fail there is often that special look—it must be in his head. Some patients have even been told this more or less directly by their physician and offered a referral for counseling. Not infrequently, a man will begin to believe that it is in his head and feel even more embarrassed, an emotional reaction that is readily experienced when it comes to conditions of the reproductive organs. Believe that it is definitely not in your head and it results directly from your vasectomy.

Symptoms typically experienced include pain on one or both sides that is either localized to a specific area or experienced as more diffuse. Radiation of the pain through-out the scrotal area and even to the back can occur, the latter expression often indicating greater damage and creating the possibility of it being misdiagnosed as kidney pain. Whatever pain is felt with PVPS, it can be worsened by activities and we are not talking about horseback riding. Commonly, there is pain accompanying sexual arousal that worsens during ejaculation. The pain can be sharp and immediate or build gradually with sexual stimulation. Pain in the epidiidymis or testicle frequently occurs after ejaculating. Now that is certainly a great form of birth control—make sex so painful you refrain from having it.

As a pain entity PVPS is about as clear as they come, falling just short of a knife sticking out of the back, which very few physicians would fail to diagnose. Rarely are the testicles of adult males painful, assuming there has been no injury. Simply inquiring whether or not the patient has suffered any injury will quickly eliminate this possibility. Even testicular cancer rarely presents with pain. Given the limited conditions promoting testicular pain in men and a history of vasectomy, it is reasonable to connect these two occurrences. Why this linkage is often not made is a mystery, but part of the problem is the adherence of urologists and other physicians providing vasectomies to the party line—Vasectomy is a "safe and simple procedure."

Regulating medical organizations despite legal actions against providers of vasectomy also seem to miss what is going on in the world of urology. I focus on urologists primarily because vasectomy and PVPS is their domain, much as schizophrenia is within the realm of psychiatry, and as such they must accept responsibility for letting the wider medical community and patients be fully aware of what changes occur following that so-called "safe and simple procedure." They must also make all concerned aware of how these changes can result in severe lifelong pain that may arise at any time. Of course this would not sell many vasectomies.

A problem that urologists who are interested in spreading the accurate word encounter is that the actual incidence—number of new cases—of PVPS is still unclear despite it being recognized as an entity in the seventies. Ajay Nangia, Jonathan Myles, and Anthony Thomas in their 2000 study—Vasectomy Reversal For The Post-Vasectomy Pain Syndrome: A Clinical And Histological Evaluation— published in The Journal Of Urology, state that the incidence is unclear partially due to the vague definition, pain threshold differences, psychological factors, and the fact that not all late complications represent PVPS.

There is also the all important issue of how long after vasectomy you evaluate men for PVPS given that it can arise at any time and is frequently misdiagnosed, particularly when a lot of time has elapsed since the vasectomy. Add to this list the embarrassment many men feel at coming forward for anything less than severe pain, and the often non-supportive reaction if they do, and it is extremely difficult to accurately say how common it is. Not surprisingly, reported incidence rates vary from less than 5% to over 50%!

If you went for a vaccination and your physician in-formed you that there is a 5% to over 50% chance of severe lifelong pain in your arm resulting from injecting the vaccine, I doubt you would say, Fine. Most would head for the door. Information regarding how common and persistent pain following vasectomy is, began appearing in the late seventies when Schmidt (1979) reported that of 154 men with sperm granulomas after vasectomy 83 (53%) experienced intense pain and 63 (41%) required surgery. When this report is combined with the knowledge that sperm granulomas are found not just on one but both sides in approximately 50% of men with vasectomies performed more than 10 years earlier, it is clear that pain from sperm granulomas alone is quite common. Of course, some researchers believe that the presence of sperm granulomas allows pressure to vent, thereby reducing the incidence of PVPS. Edward Shapiro and Sherman Silber (1979) found that none of the severed vas deferens with sperm granulomas became painful. They described patients with sperm granulomas on one side suffering pain only on the side without sperm granulomas. However, this evaluation was done 1 month following vasectomy, so the results could well have changed later when fibrous tissue formed trapping nerves.

Considering that vasectomy is the second most common surgical procedure performed on men, circumcision being the most common, it is impressive how there are so few studies following-up on the long-term complication rate. McMahon and fellow researchers—Chronic Testicular Pain Following Vasectomy—attempted a postal survey or telephone interview with 253 patients 4 years after their vasectomy. Of the 253 patients 72 could not be located and a further 9 failed to reply. The remaining 172 (68%) of the sample were assessed. The average age of the patients was 34 years. The postal questionnaire consisted of the following questions:

1. Are you aware of any differences in intercourse since your operation?   Yes/No

2. Do you get any discomfort in the penis or the testicles before, during or after intercourse?
   Yes/No

3. A few men who have had vasectomies find that they get occasional discomfort in the testicles. Do you?

   Never have any discomfort in the testicles.

   Get occasional discomfort which does not trouble you.

   Have occasional discomfort which is a nuisance.

   Have pain in the testicles which is bad enough to effect your way of life.

4. Do you ever experience any swelling in or behind your testicles?

No

Yes—occasionally

Yes—frequently

Yes—permanently

5. If you have had pain or swelling following your operation please indicate how long after the operation you first noticed it:

Pain_____

Swelling_____

The results of McMahon and fellow researchers are very informative. 56 of the 172 patients (33%) developed chronic testicular discomfort, mainly on one side. Of these men, 26, or 15% of the total 172 considered the discomfort to be a problem, whereas 30 (18%) did not. The pain was a dull ache in some cases and a sharp severe pain in others. 11 (6%) reported swelling in the scrotum. Discomfort or pain during intercourse occurred in 9 (5%) of the men who responded. Amazingly, no more than 9 sought medical help and only 2 were operated on! Clearly physicians must directly ask vasectomized patients about pain in the testicular region and not expect the information to be volunteered.

Flaws in the questionnaire used by these researchers could even have reduced the reporting of pain. Question 3 is worded inadequately in that it indicates—a few men—which suggests to readers that discomfort following vasectomy is not all that common. Wishing to avoid being lumped into a small category of sorry cases several of those who were suffering might have restrained their opinions and limited the severity of discomfort reported. The wording—occasional discomfort—also minimizes the problem because some respondents with pain might conceivable have thought the question was only assessing discomfort and not actual pain unless it was bad enough to effect their way of life, leading them to respond inaccurately.

Still another flaw with question 3 is that the response options jump from—Have occasional discomfort which is a nuisance, all the way to—Have pain in the testicles which is bad enough to affect your way of life. Only extreme ongoing pain would significantly impair way of life. A response option prior to this might have been—Ongoing discomfort or pain in the area of the testicles. In addition, the focus in the questionnaire is on the testicles, leading some to exclude pain within the scrotum but outside the testicle. With these changes the amount of reported pain would likely have been higher.

Choe and Kirkemo—Questionnaire-Based Outcomes Study Of Nononcological Post-Vasectomy Complications—reported in The Journal of Urology in 1996 noted that the incidence of post-vasectomy complications, such as chronic scrotal pain, and the impact on quality of life is not well studied or well known. A survey containing 154 questions designed to address post-vasectomy complications, the incidence of chronic scrotal pain, and the effects of such pain on quality of life, was mailed to 470 patients. 182 (38.7%) returned completed questionnaires. The average follow-up time was 52 months or just over 4 years, and the average age was 40 years.

Chronic scrotal pain occurred in 34 (19%) of patients. An additional 12 (7%) were diagnosed with epididymitis, which as we have seen is often the misdiagnosis of PVPS. Combining these values 46 or 25% of respondents experienced ongoing pain. Of the 34 patients they found with chronic scrotal pain 24 (71%) described the pain as an occasional and not troublesome, while 6 (18%) considered it a minor nuisance. Only 4 patients (2%) stated that the pain had an adverse impact on the quality of life, with it restricting physical activity for 2 patients, and creating pain during sex for the other two. The questionnaire is not included with the article so it is not clear how the phrasing of questions might have influenced the reporting of more severe pain.

Going postal again, Ahmed, Rasheed, White and Shaikh—The Incidence Of Post-Vasectomy Chronic Testicular Pain And The Role Of Nerve Stripping (Denervation) Of The Spermatic Cord In Its Management—published in the British Journal Of Urology in 1997, produced a response rate of 70% with the average age of the respondents 36 years (range 25 to 55 years) and an average time since vasectomy of 19 months (range 8 to 39 months). Of the 396 respondents 108 or 27% reported some testicular pain after their vasectomy. For 20 of these men, or 5% of all respondents, the pain persisted beyond the recovery period following surgery. Analgesics were required to relieve the pain for 33 or 8% of the 396 respondents, 14 or 3.5% had to take time off from work due to the pain, and 40 patients or 10% of the 396 complained of pain during intercourse. The pain arose between 1 and 3 months following vasectomy for 45.4% of those experiencing pain and between 3 and 6 months for an additional 32.4% of pain sufferers.

The McMahon and Choe & Kirkemo studies only used an average follow-up time since vasectomy of 4 years, while the Ahmed study used an even shorter time frame. When pain arises from sperm granulomas the time frame can be over ten years given how it takes that long for these lesions to develop on both sides. Long-term follow-up is provided in a study by Manikandan, Srirangam, Pearson and Collins—Early And Late Morbidity After Vasectomy: A Comparison Of Chronic Scrotal Pain At 1 And 10 Years—published in BJU International in 2004. Men vasectomized 10 years or 1 year prior to the study were asked to complete a questionnaire, and those reporting pain a Visual Analog Scale (VAS) to grade the intensity. In the 10 year group 13.8% of the patients had a new onset of scrotal pain of some nature, other than that arising right after surgery, compared to

16.8% in the 1year group, figures that are statistically similar.

Regarding severity of pain, 4.3% in the 10 year group had a VAS over 5 indicating severe pain and 5.9% in the 1 year group had a similar VAS score. Pain was aggravated by sexual activity in some but not all of the men. Their questionnaire, included with the article, appears well designed and very comprehensive. They address the issue of pain severity in terms of both frequency and intensity. First, "Does the pain or discomfort occur, Everyday, Every other day, Once a week, Once a month" and second, "Please mark on the scale below what best describes your pain (scale runs from 0 to 10, the further you mark to your right the more severe the pain)—No pain (0) to Worst pain ever experienced (10)." Manikandan and colleagues conclude that ongoing scrotal pain after vasectomy is more common than previously believed affecting at least 1 in 7, or approximately 14%, of patients! They advise that all patients must receive appropriate counseling prior to vasectomy.

The vasectomy literature tends to diminish the suffering from PVPS. For example, Cory Christiansen and Jay Sandlow in their excellent article (2003) on the early, intermediate, and late post-vasectomy changes mention that only a small percentage of post-vasectomy patients (less than 10%) develop PVPS. Here we have a commonly performed procedure that results in chronic, which is to say never ending, and not infrequently severe pain for perhaps 10% to 15% of vasectomized men based on the studies reviewed. Add concerns such as treatment for the condition is expensive and only available to the financially well-to-do in most countries, non-existent in third world countries, and frequently does not cure the problem, and I would say anything over a fraction of 1% is far too large a percentage. However, if the party line is maintained that it is a "safe and simple procedure" any negative results will tend to be downplayed.

Almost every urologist will encounter several PVPS patients during their career, and grapple with the best way to deal with these patients. Those lacking money or good medical coverage might truly be out in the cold. Men in third world countries are unlikely to even find out what is wrong with them let alone receive any remotely useful treatment for the problem. I will state it now—Enough is enough, the party line has to go and vasectomy needs to be viewed as flawed both theoretically and practically, such that severe damage to the vas, epididymis, efferent ducts, and even testicles invariably results from the procedure. This damage to the reproductive organs represents the massive portion of the iceberg residing below the surface with Post-Vasectomy Pain Syndrome comprising the proverbial tip of the iceberg, and a tip that can be very sharp indeed.

POSSIBLE MECHANISMS OF PAIN

Now that we know tampering with the natural state of male reproductive anatomy is not such a good idea, you might be wondering why some men end up with pain and others do not. As Shapiro and Silbert way back in 1979 mentioned, the question should not be why some men have pain but why more do not. As is often the case, why, is a difficult question to answer accurately, and in the case of Post-Vasectomy Pain Syndrome there might be different mechanisms involved making the problem more of a cluster of vasectomy after effects rather than just one specific problem.

Perhaps it is best to start with what PVPS is not. Many physicians assume that an infection is responsible for the pain and tenderness experienced by their patient. The 20 patients in Selikowitz and Schned's study (1985) were referred to the researchers for chronic epididymitis (basically an inflamed epididymis) 5 to 7 years after vasectomy. At least 6 weeks of antibiotic therapy provided by other physicians was not helpful. Initial investigations of the urine and prostate fluid from these men failed to find any infection. Treatment for 18 of their patients consisted of surgically removing the epididymis and part of the vas— epididymovasectomy (try saying that even once). Despite severe disruption of the epididymis in all 18 cases no bacteria or fungus grew with thorough attempts to culture such organisms from the removed samples, providing clear evidence that infection was not the culprit.

BACKPRESSURE & DISTENSION:

Moving to what might be responsible for the pain there are several of the usual suspects in cases of seemingly unexplained pain. One of these is backpressure and distension, in this case transmitted through the vas, epididymis, efferent ducts, and even the testicle. As Shafik (1996) in his study of pressure and electrical activity changes in the vas following vasectomy demonstrated, there is a marked increase in pressure within the vas on the testicular side following vasectomy. He suggests that distension resulting from backpressure interferes with the electrical activity of the vas responsible for effective movement of sperm. The regular pacesetter potentials are disrupted and the stronger action potentials vanish.

Next in-line, moving backwards, the epididymis clearly experiences backpressure effects. Selikowitz and Schned found dilated and sperm packed tubules. Pardanani, Patil, and Pawar (1976) discovered swelling, distension, and fullness with whitish material in some ducts. Jarvis and Dubbins (1989) noted enlargement of the epididymis with cyst formation. Likewise, the efferent ducts suffer with diameter increases of 2 to 4 times their original size. Backpressure also impacts on the testicle with resulting increases in the thickness of the seminiferous tubules and increased area within them.

While it is clear that backpressure produces dilation and distension throughout the entire system, the amount of discomfort from this is not so clear. The backpressure changes described occur routinely following vasectomy and start immediately. Pain often occurs several years after vasectomy strongly implying that the changes resulting directly from backpressure are in and of themselves insufficient to trigger the pain of PVPS. However, the possibility exists that it takes several years for accumulated changes to exceed adaptive capacity and produce pain.

ESCAPING SPERM & SPERM GRANULOMAS:

Another possible candidate for chief pain inducing mechanism is extravasation of sperm and the formation of sperm granulomas. Selikowitz and Schned noted that a unique feature of PVPS was sperm extravasation from the epididymis with or without inflammation. This occurred in 9 of the 20 epididymal specimens examined. Leakage of sperm often produces the sperm granulomas found in 7 of the 20 samples examined by Selikowitz and Schned. Schmidt (1979) described these sperm granulomas as asymptomatic or symptomatic, a nice way of saying without or with pain. The former have a stabilizing layer of epithelial cells allowing inflammation to subside. Painful sperm granulomas, on the other hand, have a wall of inflammatory cells.

Of all the researchers, Schmidt draws attention to the pain potential of sperm granulomas. He found that of 154 vasectomy patients with sperm granulomas of the vas that he encountered over 22 years, 71 had asymptomatic ones discovered at the time of vas reversal surgery, while 83 had painful ones. Of the 83, 20 experienced symptom resolution without assistance, and the remaining 63 required surgery. Of course there were many vasectomized men over the 22-year observation period with aymptomatic sperm granulomas that did not come to his attention given the lack of pain and absence of reversal surgery.

Interestingly, it appears that sperm granulomas can actually reduce the likelihood of PVPS! Shapiro and Silber (1979) found that 97% of vas deferens where an open-ended technique was applied developed sperm granulomas, but none of the patients developed pain. They discovered in their closed-ended vasectomy patients that tenderness in the epididymis was more common when a sperm granuloma failed to form at the vasectomy site. William Moss—A Comparison Of Open-End Versus Closed-End Vasectomies: A Report On 6220 Cases—published in Contraception 1992, compared 3,139 patients with open-ended vasectomies to 3,081 with closed-ended vasectomies. PVPS, described as persistent congestive epididymitis, developed in 2% of those with open-ended vasectomy but 6% of those receiving a closed-ended vasectomy.

With 97% of open-ended vasectomies producing sperm granulomas at the vasectomy site and only 2% developing PVPS, sperm granulomas cannot be held as a prime suspect. A lack of sperm granulomas might actually increase the probability of PVPS. For example, Chen and Ball (1991) only detected 4 epididymal sperm granulomas of the 15 epididymides removed to treat chronic pain. In the case of a closed-ended vasectomy, sperm and associated secretions vent forming a sperm granuloma once the immune system detects the never before encountered sperm. Open-ended vasectomies allow the sperm and fluids to drain and virtually guarantee an immune reaction to the sperm, resulting in the formation of a sperm granuloma. While the evidence certainly seems more favorable for open-ended vasectomies there are reasons for caution. Although most sperm granulomas are not painful some can be very painful and encouraging their formation is questionable.

By exposing sperm to the immune system antisperm antibodies are more likely to form with an open-ended vasectomy, at least theoretically. Nancy Alexander and Stanwood Schmidt—Incidence Of Antisperm Antibody Levels And Granulomas In Men-reported in Fertility And Sterility in 1977—obtained blood samples from 77 men prior to vasectomy reversal. Vasectomies had been performed 1 to 20 years earlier. 67% of the men with granulomas had sperm immobilizing antibodies compared to 48% of the men with no granulomas. There is concern that these antisperm antibodies adversely affect other organs of the body as they circulate around. There is also the issue of their influence on the epididymis.

INFLAMMTION & FIBROSIS:

Moving away from the controversy of antisperm antibodies to the more clearly defined results of vasectomy we need to focus on another of the usual pain suspects—inflammation and fibrosis. As part of the healing process and reaction to injury the body produces hard scar-like tissue, a process referred to as fibrosis, to contrast it with the formation of hard connective tissue occurring during routine growth. In their study, The Vulnerability of the Vas Deferens, Shandling and Janik (1981) found that simply clamping the vas of rats could produce muscle disruption and fibrosis.

The unique architecture of the vas with it being the only tubular structure where the diameter of the lumen is less than the thickness of the wall makes it vulnerable to injury. The thick muscle layers can easily become disrupted with an insult more minor than vasectomy triggering fibrosis. Propulsion of sperm dependent on the smooth muscle of the vas suffers, sperm accumulates, and some of it extravasates. Shandling and Janik found cysts from which fluid spread between the muscle layers. With more extensive damage comes increased inflammation and fibrosis worsening the whole scenario.

Fibrosis also occurs in the epididymis and testicles. Chen and Ball reported fibrosis often with entrapment of nerves in the epididymis. McMahon and fellow researchers (1992) performed ultrasound on 27 patients who had undergone vasectomy, 14 with chronic discomfort. Of the 14 patients experiencing pain 4 had multiple epididymal cysts, both sides. Epididymal cysts can result in inflammation and a fibrotic response. Jarrow and fellow researchers (1985) found fibrosis in the space between the seminiferous tubules of the testicles. Of particular interest is the finding that fibrosis within the testicles following vasectomy is highly related to inability to regain fertility following reversal surgery.

A common reaction to vasectomy, sperm granulomas are not to be excluded from the realm of fibrosis. The symptomatic sperm granulomas described by Schmidt (1979) have a wall of inflammatory cells with fibrous tissue forming around the wall to contain the inflammation. Schmidt noted that due to the proximity of the vas to other structures of the spermatic cord, the nerves and blood vessels can become incorporated into the walls of the sperm granuloma.

NERVE ENTRAPMENT:

With fibrosis any nerves thus incorporated would be effectively cemented in place. Upon even light touch the trapped sensory nerve is compressed, as it is when a bolus of sperm reaches it during ejaculation. Pain during intercourse and ejaculation also occurs because with arousal and ejaculation muscles elevate the testis, pushing sperm granulomas against the external ring of the inguinal canal through which the vas, blood vessels, and nerves pass into the body. Pain with sexual arousal can be so severe that some men refrain from intercourse, a pleasant result of vasectomy to be sure. I wonder how many physicians performing vasectomies stress this point to their patients.

A concern related to nerve entrapment is whether or not nerves grow into the tissue. Actual nerve proliferation was not found in the research conducted by Nangia, Myles, and Thomas (2000). However, Reinhard Pabst, Otmar Martin and Herbert Lippert—Is The Low Fertility Rate After Vasovasostomy Caused By Nerve Resection During Vasectomy? (Fertility And Sterility, 1979), found a large number of nerves running parallel to the vas that are easily cut or damaged during a vasectomy. Cut nerves might theoretically grow into fibrous tissue.

Pain without sensory nerve involvement is like hating the sound of screaming babies when you have been completely deaf since birth. Nerves have to be involved somehow. Apparently sleeping through nerve anatomy courses, advocates of vasectomy seem to have forgotten that there is an extremely rich nerve supply along the spermatic cord, including the spermatic sympathetic plexus containing the sensory nerves for the testes. With so many nerves and other structures compacted into a cord-like structure it is not surprising that nerves can be trapped in fibrous tissue or somehow irritated by it, particularly if cut during the vasectomy. Recall that Chen and Ball found nerves around the vasectomy site and epididymis solidly encased in fibrous tissue with distortion, angulation, and inflammatory cell involvement! Trapping, reconfiguring, and igniting an inflammatory response in a sensory nerve has got to hurt, no rocket science here folks.

Fibrosis is a common reaction to vasectomy and can occur at virtually any location—vas, epididymis, efferent ducts, and testicle. The most common factor associated with fibrosis is extravasation, or in other words leakage, of sperm into the tubule walls and beyond. Once normal mechanisms to reabsorb sperm concentrated in the epididymis and efferent ducts are overwhelmed, specialized so-called phagocytic cells enter the various tubular structures to assist. The buildup of these cells with digested sperm can initiate an inflammatory reaction that likely compromises the integrity of the tubular walls beyond what simple pressure effects account for. Eventually sperm pass out of the space inside and into the walls. If the process occurs very slowly and is limited, a stabilizing layer of epithelial cells can resolve the inflammation. In many cases the speed and extent of sperm leakage is such that an inflammatory response persists and fibrous tissue is generated to contain the inflammatory process. A symptomatic sperm granuloma is frequently how this manifests, but any significant inflammatory process in any part of the system can result in fibrosis. It is even likely that the rare cases of infectious agent involvement produce inflammation leading to fibrosis that can entrap a sensory nerve. While different theories exist as to why pain occurs, any way it is viewed, nerve involvement is present, and very much so. All of the usual pain suspects almost certainly have as their final pain pathway nerve entrapment or irritation. From this it follows that any effective intervention must correct nerve entrapment but more on this intriguing topic later on.

Two unique conditions related somewhat to PVPS— genitofemoral and ilioinguinal entrapment neuralgia—are very revealing. Without getting into the highly complex nerve anatomy the genitofemoral and ilioinguinal nerves are two important nerves in the general region of the groin. With surgery for removal of an appendix or inguinal hernia repair (hernia is protrusion of tissue into an area it should not be, such as bowel tissue into the inguinal canal connecting the scrotum to the pelvic cavity) these nerves or a branch of one of them can become encased in fibrous tissue. Patients experience intermittent or chronic pain and/or burning sensations typically not responding well to most interventions. Not infrequently they are told that the pain is in their head. Starling and fellow researchers—Diagnosis and Treatment of Genitofemoral and Ilioinguinal Entrapment Neuralgia—published in Surgery 1987, found that 88% of their ilioinguinal neuralgia patients and 77% of their genitofemoral neuralgia patients were pain free following removal of the trapped portion of the nerve! Impressive evidence of the role that fibrous tissue can play in chronic pain syndromes of the genital region, and how surgery directed at removing nerves from fibrous tissue can be highly successful.

OPEN-ENDED VERSUS
CLOSED-ENDED VASECTOMY

Ideally, there should be no vasectomies performed given the inherent risk of Post-Vasectomy Pain Syndrome, but if they are to be offered is one basic technique superior to the other? In the early years of vasectomy it was apparently fairly common to leave the testicular end open, but concerns that this might increase the risk of spontaneous recanalization (natural reconnection of the cut vas following vasectomy) and pregnancy, began appearing as early as the late 1940's, such as O'Conor's Anastomosis Of Vas Deferens After Purposeful Division For Sterility published in the Journal Of The American Medical Association in 1948. These concerns ushered in a period that we are currently still in dominated by closed-ended vasectomies.

Michel Labrecque and fellow researchers—Effectiveness And Complications Associated With 2 Vasectomy Occlusion Techniques—published in The Journal Of Urology in 2002, compared 2,040 men vasectomized with the closed-ended method and 1,721 men vasectomized with the open-ended method. For the former group they applied a strategy called clipping and excision whereby clips are placed approximately 1 cm apart on the vas and the section between them is cut out. Their open-ended technique consisted of first, cutting the vas and sealing 1 cm of the abdominal end with thermal cautery (burning it essentially), and secondly, interposing the connective tissue sheath found around the vas over the abdominal end. This technique is referred to as cautery and interposition.

Failures, confirmed or possible, involved sperm appearing in the ejaculate well past the time frame and number of ejaculations required for it to clear from the abdominal end following a vasectomy. The failure rate was 8.7% for the closed-ended and .3% for the open-ended or 7.6% versus .1% when confirmed cases only were considered. For the last 2 study years there was not a single confirmed or possible failure with the open-ended technique applied! This is an absolutely amazing result when we consider that the open-ended vasectomy method has been largely rejected in favor of the closed-ended method due to unwanted pregnancies concerns.

The term open-ended is a misnomer as there would never be a vasectomy performed that is truly open-ended. One side of the vas is always sealed off. This name invites the perception that open-ended vasectomy will result in a higher rate of unwanted pregnancies. In fact, the opposite is true as evidenced by the results of Michel Labrecque's study—Sperm are much more likely to appear in the ejaculate with closed-ended vasectomy. But how could this possibly be?

The culprit appears to be the seemingly innocent but never neutral sperm granuloma. As Sherman Silber mentions in Reversal Of Vasectomy And The Treatment Of Male Infertility (1981), spontaneous recanalization occurs when sperm leaks out through the cut testicular end of the vas and swims through the connective tissue, grinding a pathway to the other side. According to Ajay Nangia and fellow researchers (2000) sperm granulomas are almost always associated with the proliferation of ductules within the walls, referred to as vasitis nodosum when noninflammatory. Schmidt back in 1979 identified 4 cases of the testicular end reconnecting with the prostate end, and all were associated with a sperm granuloma. Mostly, this passage of sperm results in a low sperm count, poor motility of the sperm, and in some cases the route will scar down and seal off, but the capacity to impregnate does exist. Schmidt also recorded cases of tubules connecting to the skin surface appearing as painful recurrent "pimples" that would burst, drain, and then close, or as a persistent wet spot. These occurrences probably diminish romance contributing a further dimension to birth control.

Sperm granulomas at the closed-ended vasectomy site essentially provide a connective tissue conduit, and remain on the same tissue plane as the abdominal end of the vas. As Michel Labrecque indicates, open-ended vasectomy with connective tissue interposition of the abdominal end of the vas, separates the tissue planes greatly reducing the likelihood of spontaneous recanalization. Studies reporting higher rates of spontaneous recanalization with the open-ended method have not included connective tissue interposition. Any sperm granuloma that forms after open-ended vasectomy with tissue interposition of the abdominal side occurs on a different plane than the prostate end of the vas and cannot form a conduit.

In regards to unwanted pregnancies open-ended vasectomies, despite the name, are clearly superior to closed-ended, but what about adverse symptoms. Larecque found that the rate of painful granulomas at the vasectomy site, noninfectious inflammation of the vas, epididymis or testicle, and pain without a clear cause were similar with closed-ended and open-ended vasectomies. Comparing 3,867 men vasectomized by the closed-ended method to 4,330 open-ended vasectomy recipients, Australian researchers Bruce Errey and Ian Edwards—Open-Ended Vasectomy: An Assessment—published in Fertility and Sterility, 1986, assessed the number of men returning for complications identified as either epididymal congestion or granuloma. Sexual intercourse or minor trauma often triggered sudden discomfort leading to the visit. Men in the open-ended vasectomy group were significantly less likely to return to the clinic during the first year following their vasectomy, than were men in the closed-ended group for either problem. Only 1 case of spontaneous recanalization of the vas occurred in the open-ended group whereas 3 transpired in the closed-ended group.

In a similar study William Moss (1992) reviewed records of 3,081 men who received closed-ended vasectomy and 3,139 with open-ended vasectomy. In each series 300 cases were evaluated for congestive epididymtis. Most cases were triggered by sexual intercourse or minor trauma as with the Errey and Edwards study. The incidence was significantly higher in the closed-ended group than in the open-ended group—6% versus 2% respectively. Some non-tender sperm granulomas were noted in both groups.

One of the intriguing findings from both studies is the presence of sperm granulomas in the open-ended vasectomy recipients. Sperm granulomas vent high pressure arising from blocked outflow of sperm filled secretions from the testicles. If the cut end of the vas on the testicular side actually remains open, drainage into the scrotal area should prevent any significant pressure increase, thereby eliminating the defensive response of sperm granuloma formation. Once again the unique structure of the vas deferens—thick wall and narrow lumen—plays a role by increasing the likelihood that the cut ends will scar over transforming an open-ended vasectomy into a closed-ended one with all the associated backpressure effects. Errey and Edward found that most patients in the open-ended group returning due to symptomatic sperm granulomas did so after the first couple of months. Immediately following vasectomy scarring is minimal and then increases as part of the long-range response to the trauma. Aside from scarring over, backpressure can result from impaired propulsion of sperm and secretions due to interference with the electrical activity of the vas resulting from the vasectomy.

Even if the testicular end of the vas remains open sperm granulomas will form, because the immune system detects exiting sperm, and launches both cell-based and so-called humoral (antibody) responses to the foreign bodies. The cell-based response initiates sperm granuloma formation. Hence, sperm granulomas are to be expected with open-ended vasectomy. In support of this proposition, Edward Shapiro and Sherman Silber (1979) found that 97% of patients receiving an open-ended vasectomy in one series and 100% in another series developed a sperm granuloma at the vasectomy site. No mention was made of the occurrence rate in the epididymis. It is not reasonable to assume that 97% to 100% of open-ended vasectomies scarred over, and hence sperm granulomas must have formed without any build up in hydrostatic pressure! Most of the sperm granulomas were small (3mm or less), decreased in size over 2 to 4 months, and were nontender. Perhaps sperm granulomas that develop in the absence of hydrostatic pressure are more likely to be of the asymptomatic type described by Schmidt. Sperm granulomas venting high pressure might be more likely to be of the inflammatory type and entrap nerves leading to chronic pain.

So far it all seems good news for the open-ended method, but there is a potential disadvantage in that the cautery and interposition technique is more complicated to perform than closed-ended techniques, leading to a higher rate of early complication. In particular, hematomas (localized masses of extravasated blood) occur more with the open-ended method—1.6% compared to .5% in the closed-ended group in the Michel Labrecque research study. He found that most were small and did not require surgical drainage. The risk of noninfectious pain due to granulomas or inflammation of the vas or testes, were similar for both groups—4.1% open-ended and 3.5% closed-ended. In Moss's study there were 2 hematomas in the open-ended group, neither requiring drainage, and none in the closed-ended group.

In reviewing the evidence it is difficult not to conclude that the "open-ended" method is superior to the closed-ended method, both in terms of reduced risk of unwanted pregnancy and diminished rates of undesirable effects on the testicular end of the vas, epididymis, efferent ducts, and testicle. Fewer adverse affects translate into fewer painful sperm granulomas and other sources of PVPS, even though the risk is definitely not eliminated. Obviously, with any vasectomy trauma and scarring can occur resulting in nerve entrapment and chronic pain. The greater technical difficulty encountered with interposing the connective tissue sheath over the abdominal end of the vas, increases the likelihood of damage and scarring as suggested by the higher rate of hematomas with this technique. The current practice of physicians with limited training and experience performing vasectomies must then end, and only those with advanced training and significant surgical experience be permitted to perform the procedure. Such a change is not likely to go over well with those who enjoy the economic return for this simple elective procedure. Perhaps increased payments arising from litigation based on the evidence presented here might discourage all but the most competent from offering vasectomy to patients.

TREATMENTS FOR POST-VASECTOMY PAIN SYNDROME

Post-Vasectomy Pain Syndrome is a chronic condition meaning that it must persist beyond 6, or at least 3, months following vasectomy. Certain factors might aggravate it, such as sexual intercourse and ejaculation, and it might vary in intensity, but it does not disappear on its own. Following vasectomy swelling of the epididymis with some discomfort or pain is quite common, likely due to the largely unavoidable trauma of the procedure. Within days or weeks, sometimes with the aid of ice packs, anti-inflammatory medication and other conservative procedures the swelling settles. By 3 months this problem should be resolved. Long-range pain that can appear years after the vasectomy is what requires more aggressive treatment.

Some surgeons state that PVPS can be treated effectively by surgery, a statement that can be dangerously inaccurate. Although surgery can be used to correct what surgery caused in the first place, hopefully the income aspects are not missed on readers, the various surgical approaches only enjoy a limited success rate and ongoing pain is not uncommon. In a worst case scenario the testicle will have to be removed—orchiectomy—and then the remaining testicle will become painful. One of the fascinating things, although not necessarily to suffers of PVPS, is how pain is sometimes only felt on one side, as if the stronger pain signal overrides the weaker pain signal. Following vasectomy the left side might be the only one producing pain. After surgical correction, the pain signal on the right side can be heard and that side becomes painful. It appears that vasectomy is a "safe and simple procedure" only to the truly simple of mind.

I will state it now for all to remember—No procedure will work in the long run unless the fibrosis and nerves trapped within or irritated by it are removed. The actual procedure does not appear as important as does managing this one crucial aspect. This consideration appears to be one of the main reasons for varying success rates by different surgeons and for different techniques. A technically perfect reversal procedure might fail relative to a less than ideal one that succeeds in clearing out all the affected nerves.

Medicine based treatments for PVPS do not work. Often patients have been through several courses of antibiotics, anti-inflammatory agents, and techniques like ice packs to no avail. A 2-3 month course of Ciprofloxacin, or equivalent antibiotic, might help in the event of a prostate infection that has been unleashed, but resolution of PVPS is unlikely because an infection of this severity often results in fibrosis. Some clinicians try injecting a local pain killer and/or anti-inflammatory agent right into the painful region. This procedure can provide temporary relief until surgery and might unmask the weaker pain signal on the other side. I suggest that as part of the treatment plan for PVPS, surgeons should inject a strong local anesthetic right into the heart of the painful area to determine whether or not any pain is experienced on the other side. If so the odds are high that the patient will experience pain on the remaining side after treating the primary side. It should be noted by both patients and physicians that local injections can be very detrimental because they induce further trauma and fibrosis that can in turn lead to even more pain.

Surgical interventions for PVPS include transforming a closed-ended vasectomy into an open-ended, removal of a tender sperm granuloma, reversing the vasectomy, stripping the nerves from the spermatic cord, removal of the epididymis, and orchiectomy.

CLOSED-ENDED TO OPEN-ENDED VASECTOMY:

The simplest approach to treating Post-Vasectomy Pain Syndrome is transforming a closed-ended vasectomy into an open-ended one. Sperm granulomas will still form, but ongoing pressure induced drainage of testicular secretions into inflamed sperm granulomas might be replaced with free drainage into the scrotal cavity. If a blockage within the epididymis has already formed it is unlikely that a revised vasectomy will work. Neither is it likely to resolve the pain unless all trapped or irritated nerves are removed during the procedure. Care should be taken to preserve as much of the vas as possible since the presence of longer sections can assist in the success of reversal procedures.

REMOVAL OF PAINFUL SPERM GRANULOMAS:

Schmidt (Spermatic Granuloma: An Often Painful Lesion) noted over a 22-year period, 63 cases of painful sperm granuloma requiring surgery. The most common complaint was a painful mass at the cut end of the vasectomy, at times large enough to be a tumor—Frequently, vasectomized men feel a lump and wonder if it is a tumor, adding an anxiety component to their other problems. Schmidt found that pain was frequently experienced during sexual excitement, often severe at ejaculation, such that the patient would avoid intercourse because of fear of the pain—a truly effective form of birth control! The pain sometimes radiated to the flank, a severe form of the condition. These patients were commonly diagnosed as having kidney stones leading to further investigations for this problem.

Examining these painful sperm granulomas under the microscope Schmidt discovered that the wall incorporated surrounding nerves and blood vessels. When the granuloma is compressed by a bolus of sperm reaching it during ejaculation, or the muscles that elevate the testicles during ejaculation press it against the external ring where the spermatic cord exits the body, or inflammation affects it, the nerve is stimulated and pain arises. Schmidt removed the offending sperm granuloma in each of the 63 men to relieve their pain.

VASECTOMY REVERSAL:

Perhaps the most common method of treating PVPS is reversal of the vasectomy, either by reconnecting the severed ends of the vas together—vasovasostomy—or by reconnecting the prostate end of the vas to the epididymis—vasoepididymostomy. Impressive words but breaking them down we have "ostomy" meaning creating an opening, in this case between two hollow organs, and "vaso" referring to a vessel. The vessel here is the vas and an opening is created between the prostate side and either the testicular section of the vas or the epididymis. These operations have been devised and refined for restoration of fertility when a vasectomized man wants to conceive again. An entire class of surgical technique designed to remedy what surgery—vasectomy—caused. It is an amazing world.

Vasovasostomy is the simpler of the two reversal procedures. Quinby in 1919 performed the first successful reversal for a patient vasectomized 8 years earlier. In the early days reversals were performed without the aid of surgical microscopes and not surprisingly there was a lower success rate even with less stringent evaluation criteria. A survey by O'Conor in 1948 suggested a 35% to 40% success rate. In the seventies came the microscopic vasovasostomy with Sherman Silber popularizing the procedure.

In his classic paper—Microscopic Vasectomy Reversal—published in Fertility And Sterility in 1977, Sherman Silber described over 300 reversals with an overall success rate of 71% based on pregnancy achieved by the partner.

Silber found that the presence of sperm granulomas predicted better quality sperm in the testicular side of the vas prior to reconnection. In the absence of a sperm granuloma, length of time from the original vasectomy had a pronounced impact with low success rates after 10 years. His 2-layer technique, involving first suturing the inner mucosal layer containing the epithelial lining and then the muscle layer, has become the standard and is probably optimal for long-term success, although some surgeons use a 1-layer technique.

Since the earlier microscopic vasovasostomy research of Sherman Silber the factors accounting for a successful reversal operation have become clearer. One key factor is the skill of the surgeon with success rates increasing with more experience performing reversal operations. Harris Nagler and Michael Rotman—Predictive Parameters For Microsurgical Reconstruction—published in Urologic Clinics Of North America (2002) report that those surgeons who do not practice the technique have a 53% success rate as opposed to 89% for those who at least practice in the lab. Given the implications when treating PVPS, a surgeon's experience will be particularly important.

Other factors predictive of success include:

– Vas fluid that is watery as opposed to creamy or cloudy because the former is more likely to have viable sperm.

– A longer testicular segment of the vas to work with.

– A shorter interval from vasectomy to reversal.

Generally speaking, success rates in terms of significant numbers of motile sperm in the ejaculate (patency) and pregnancy occur in over 90% and 70% respectively when the vasectomy to reversal interval is less than 3 years, and 70% and 30% respectively if the interval is 15 years or longer.

Vasoepididymostomy, also referred to as tubulovaso-tomy, is a more technically challenging procedure due to the delicate nature of the highly coiled epididymis. Failure to detect sperm in the fluid on the testicular side of the vas suggests that there is a blockage in the epididymis and that reconnecting the ends of the vas will fail. Sherman Silber (1977) described connecting the vas to the epididymal tubule using his 2-layer method. Starting at the lower section connected to the vas (tail) the epididymis is sectioned until good quality sperm is detected indicating no blockage at this point. The blockage most often is found at the junction of the body and tail where the epididymal tubule first becomes thinned out.

The site of the blockage within the epididymis is important for the success of the procedure. Anthony Thomas— Vasoepididymostomy—published in Urologic Clinic Of North America in 1987, mentions that sperm progressively mature and gain motility as they pass through the head and body of the epididymis. The tail of the epididymis serves largely as a storage reservoir for mature sperm, having the capacity to hold over 400 million sperm! When the blockage is in the tail section success rates in terms of sperm appearing in the ejaculate and pregnancy are better and the results occur faster. The higher up that the blockage in the epididymis is, the lower the success rate and slower the appearance of motile sperm when there is success. However, even in this case patency rates of greater than 60% are achieved. In general, patency rates from 70% to 80% and pregnancy rates from 30% to 55% are achieved with vasoepididymostomy.

As technology improves success with vasectomy reversal also improves. Currently, there is a lot of research into newer methods such as bio-glues (fibrin glue) and special stents (artificial tubes in this case) to achieve an easier and less costly reversal. Innovative procedures such as connecting both testicular vas sections to one on the prostate side have been successfully performed.

All of this is good news for those wishing to regain fertility, but what about the success rates in resolving PVPS? Ajay Nangia, Jonathan Myles and Anthony Thomas (2000), reviewed the records of 13 patients who underwent reversal surgery for PVPS. Pain onset occurred from 9 days to 9 years following vasectomy with an average of 2 years, and was present on both sides in 10 cases, one-sided in the other 3. One of these 3 men previously had the vasectomy reversed on both sides due to PVPS and the pain returned on one side. The length of time between vasectomy and reversal ranged from less than 1 year to 14 years, with an average of 4.8 years. Their ages ranged from 23 to 54 with an average of 34.9. I find it truly amazing that a vasectomy would be provided to a man as young as 23.

For 9 of the men (69%) the pain resolved completely, and for the remaining 4 there was partial relief. One man was pain free for a year but the pain returned on both sides. Analysis of his ejaculate failed to reveal any sperm indicating that the reversal scarred over on both sides. The researchers evaluated the ejaculate of 7 men 1 month to 3 years after reversal, noting sperm in 6 cases, and 4 free of pain.

In a larger study, Stanley Myers, Christopher Mershon and Eugene Fuchs—Vasectomy Reversal For Treatment Of The Post-Vasectomy Pain Syndrome—published in The Journal Of Urology in 1997, described 32 patients suffering from PVPS who underwent vasovasostomy and/or vasoepididymostomy. All their patients complained of testicular pain on one or both sides, described as a constant dull ache that increased with sexual arousal, intercourse, or ejaculation. The interval from vasectomy to reversal ranged from 15 to 244 months with an average of 59 months, and the age of the patients was from 23 to 43 years with an average age of 31.

The follow-up period ranged from 3 to 102 months with an average of 29 months. Prior to being seen by Myers and colleagues 4 of the 32 men underwent removal of the epididymis and when this failed removal of the testicle. They then began experiencing pain in the remaining testicle! What a nightmare. Myer's group performed vasovasostomy on both sides for 23 of their patients, one-sided vasovasostomy for 3, vasovasostomy on one side and vasoepididymostomy on the other side in 2, vasoepididymostomy on both sides in 2, and vasoepididymostomy on only one side in 2 patients. The pain was completely or greatly decreased in 24 of their 32 patients, Unfortunately, 8 patients had persistent or recurrent pain, 5 on one side only and 2 on both sides. The remaining patient who previously had a testicle removed continued to experience pain in the single testicle.

Even though the follow-up period with Myers's study is quite good it would have been interesting to see whether or not the results persisted over the long range, because reversals often scar over producing a return to the vasectomized state. At the present time the rate of failed reversals is not well documented, or documented at all, but it is the experience of some urologists that it is substantially higher than what many would ideally hope for. There are several men who undergo 3 or even more attempts at reversal!

The patients who did not improve in Myer's study might have experienced failed reversals, resulting in sperm granulomas to vent increasing pressure with subsequent nerve entrapment or irritation. Another compatible explanation is that the offending nerves were removed inadvertently in the patients who improved and missed in those who did not. During the course of reversal operations nerves must be removed to properly expose the field and perform the necessary steps. If enough of the right nerves are cut out pain will diminish or vanish, plus be less likely to return in the event of a failed reversal involving sperm granuloma formation at the site. Hence, removal of the offending nerves both manages the current pain and reduces the likelihood of renewed pain if the vasectomy reversal fails.

REMOVAL OF OFFENDING NERVES:

Of all the methods that have been attempted to treat PVPS this one is most focused on the all-important matter of dealing with nerves that are either encased in fibrosis and/or sperm granulomas, or irritated by fibrotic changes arising from vasectomy. A logical but apparently underutilized technique involves isolating the painful region and surgically removing nerves and fibrous tissue found in the vicinity. This targets the particular pain sensation and minimizes surgery that could lead to further fibrosis and nerve entrapment or irritation.

Denervation (de means away from and nervation nerves) is a more extensive procedure along the same line. Essentially, all nerves along the spermatic cord are removed leaving only the vas and blood vessels. Ahmed, Rasheed, White, and Shaikh—The Incidence Of Post-Vasectomy Chronic Testicular Pain And The Role Of Nerve Stripping (Denervation) Of The Spermatic Cord In Its Management— described 17 patients who underwent spermatic cord denervation. Their patients ranged from 34 to 60 years of age, with a average of 43 years, and they presented with pain from 1 to 26 years after their vasectomy, average 6 years. Pain was present for at least a year, was felt during intercourse and required time off from work. For 9 the pain was experienced on both sides while the other 8 only felt it on the one side. Interestingly, the researchers also identified 14 patients who required analgesics (pain relief medication) for their pain but were not operated on.

Spermatic cord denervation was highly successful in this study with 13 of the 17 patients experiencing complete pain relief and 4 an 80% reduction in their pain symptoms. They were checked at intervals of 3 months and although the follow-up period is not specified it appears that it is in the range of 2 to 4 years. In a similar study, Levine and Matkov—Microsurgical Denervation Of The Spermatic Cord As

A Primary Surgical Treatment Of Chronic Orchialgia—published in the Journal Of Urology in 2001, reported 76% pain free and 9.1% partial pain relief. They divided the main nerve (ilioinguinal) and buried the abdominal end under muscle to prevent reactive fibrosis. The smaller nerves were dissected out with removal of the previous vasectomy site in case nerves were entrapped. The vas was severed at another site to maintain the vasectomized state. Unfortunately, the denervation procedure is complicated to perform and hence is not widely available.

Further support for the practice of removing entrapped nerves is the work of James Starling and colleagues (1987) who reported on patients suffering inguinal pain following various types of surgery in the region. These patients were often misdiagnosed and were sometimes considered to be neurotic or faking. The entrapped portion of the nerve (genitofemoral or ilioinguinal) was removed in 30 patients. Pathology reports indicated fibrous adhesions in 13 patients. Regarding success of the procedure, approximately 80% of their patients experienced complete pain relief although the follow-up period is not specified. They emphasized that persistent pain indicates entrapment of the neighboring sensory nerves. Compared to other surgical procedures removal of offending nerves and associated fibrous tissue does seem to have a high success rate, but longer patient follow-up periods are required to determine if the pain-free status continues.

REMOVAL OF THE EPIDIDYMIS & EFFERENT DUCTS:

Following closed-ended, and in some cases open-ended, vasectomy many changes take place in the epididymis and the efferent ducts, including thickening of the muscle layer, widening of the tubules, sperm granulomas, and fibrous tissue forming in the space between the tubules, the latter observed by Chen and Ball (1991) to actually encase nerves in some cases. Epididymal "blow-outs" occur when the tubule ruptures due to the increased pressure and breakdown of resilience. Less dramatic leakage of trapped sperm into the walls of the tubule is more common, with both processes leading to the formation of sperm granulomas that can be very painful when nerves become involved. Given the striking changes to these structures following vasectomy, it seems logical to remove the epididymis (and efferent ducts along with the epididymis) when there is chronic pain associated with tenderness in this region.

Epididymectomy (removal of the epididymis) was the treatment option selected by Stuart Selikowitz and Alan Schned (1985) for 18 patients with ongoing epididymal pain and swelling 5 to 7 years after their vasectomy, earlier diagnosed with "chronic epididymitis" (inflammation). Their discomfort was usually constant, often disabling, worsened by sexual activity, and sometimes radiated along the spermatic cord. A total of 20 epididymides were removed after the nerves and blood vessels were carefully dissected away. Along with the epididymis the vas up to the vasectomy site was removed. No infections were detected in any of the tissue samples and there were relatively few inflammatory cells when compared to infected epididymides. However, compared to normal epididymides they noted sperm extravasation into the wall of the tubule and sperm granulomas, dilation of the tubule, and sperm-packed tubules. Except for 1 patient there was complete pain relief usually within 24 hours. Unfortunately, their study did not follow patients to determine whether or not the pain returned.

Chen and Ball (1991) performed 15 epididymectomies on 10 patients with PVPS and assessed them 3 months following surgery. The outcomes were rated as good when there were no residual pain symptoms, and poor when pain and tenderness persisted. A good outcome was seen with 5 of the 10 patients, 2 with epididymectomy performed on both sides. Time since vasectomy ranged from 6 months to 10 years. Comparing their results to those of Selikowitch and Schned, they comment that the lower success rate of epididymectomy with their patients was probably due to their not excising the vas up to and including the vasectomy site, leaving some fibrosis behind as a result. While this is a plausible explanation, it could also be that the results of the two studies would be similar with the same follow-up period.

In 1996 Padmore, Norman and Miller—Analyses Of Indication For And Outcomes Of Epididymectomy— published in the Journal Of Urology, found that only 43% of their patients who underwent epididymectomy for pain were satisfied with the outcome, and suggested that patients be counseled regarding the likelihood of a poor prognosis. In another study—Epididymectomy Is An Effective Treatment For Scrotal Pain After Vasectomy—published in the BJU International in 2000, West, Leung, and Powell assessed the long-term outcome by telephone interview an average of 5.5 years after the operation. Of the 19 patients 14 (73.5%) had a good response. Those with a poor response tended to show microscopic signs of chronic inflammatory change within the epididymis. Hence, it appears that epididymectomy can be an effective treatment for PVPS but results are variable, and once again, the key factor is likely the successful removal of every nerve encased in or irritated by fibrosis. If the epididymectomy achieves this it is likely to be effective. The good results after 5 years in the study by West and colleagues is encouraging.

REMOVAL OF THE TESTICLE:

Orchiectomy should be the absolute last resort with at least a second opinion by a urologist highly experienced in vasectomy reversal procedures. Removing a testicle also removes the source of male hormones, and will prove completely useless if the patient returns complaining of pain in the remaining testicle, which is not an uncommon occurrence due to how testicular pain is frequently only experienced on the side emitting the strongest pain signal. Once the loudest signal is removed, the lesser one will be heard—the nightmare might never cease. I strongly suggest that before removal of the testicle an attempt is made by a urologist having a great deal of experience with this type of problem, to dissect out any nerves that might be either caught up in or irritated by fibrosis and/or a sperm granuloma.

COUNSELLING & INFORMED CONSENT

At first glance it might seem that counseling and informed consent are one and the same, but there are major differences between the two. Counseling provides an opportunity for the patient to examine motivations, state of mind, and relationship issues impacting on their decision. Informed consent focuses on the risks and benefits of the procedure, and also alternative options. Counseling and informed consent for vasectomy need to be treated much more rigorously than is the norm. Most prospective patients are never counseled and few receive the full story when asked to consent. Even when patients inquire about pain following the procedure they are often not informed of Post-Vasectomy Pain Syndrome, and are rarely informed of the full implications.

Given the relative simplicity of the actual operation more time should be spent on counseling and obtaining fully informed consent than on the surgery itself. Surgeons who doubt this might take heed of the comment by Gingwell, Crosby, and Carroll in their paper—Review Of The Complications And Medicolegal Implications Of Vasectomy—published in the Postgraduate Medical Journal in 2001 who state, "There can be few operations so simple to carry out under local anesthesia on an outpatient basis which carry so much potential for criticism, complaint, and allegations of incompetence."

COUNSELING:

When a person receives counseling for any given issue it is common for thoughts and feelings to arise afterwards that might well influence key decisions. Hence, counseling for vasectomy should be provided well prior to the scheduled date of the procedure, ideally a month beforehand. The man's spouse should be present for at least part of the counseling session to explore how the decision has been arrived at and the state of their relationship. However, time alone with the patient is crucial so that private concerns can be voiced freely of the partner. A month interval between counseling and vasectomy will give an opportunity for both parties to discuss issues that have arisen and reach a joint decision. Medicaid regulations in many states in the US require a 30-day waiting period between patient consent and procedure.

If the spouse desires it more than the prospective patient there might well be pressure exerted either overtly, such as indicating that ongoing sexual relations are not likely unless he gets a vasectomy, or more covertly, such as by guilt induction. Numerous examples of the latter exist—"Look at all I did for us by bearing our children," "I went through so much pain during delivery," "I don't know if I can take another child." Whenever overt or covert pressure is detected a counselor should recommend and document to the effect that vasectomy is advised against, and that alternatives have been discussed. A referral for couple counseling is strongly suggested to help sort out the issues in the relationship that might be influencing the decision to have a vasectomy. In the event that there is no spouse, there is unlikely to be a sufficient reason for having a vasectomy. In several of these cases the person has been abused during childhood and does not want children. Psychotherapy, is much more desirable than sterilization as a treatment for this type of difficulty.

In reviewing the various studies, it amazes me how many physicians seem willing to perform vasectomies on men in their twenties. People of this age are usually sorting out their direction in life and might well desire another child later on, particularly if some tragedy befalls one of their children or they enter into another relationship. Given a divorce rate of 40% to 50% and the average length of marriages around 7 years, the probability is high that many of these men will end up with a new partner who is still in her reproductive years. I strongly believe that vasectomies should never be performed on men less than 30 years of age.

Considering that the physician is selling surgery because the procedure is strictly elective and there is no urgent indication, such as eliminating pain or removing cancerous tissue, it is highly recommended that a trained individual other than the physician provide the counseling. If there is no option other than for the physician to provide it, satisfactory completion of a counseling program for sterilization approved by the relevant governing medical body should be mandatory.

The counseling session itself must include questions pertaining to the man's motivation and reasons for vasectomy, pressure exerted on the individual by others, and the current state of the marriage or relationship. One of the key rules in life is never assume anything, and nowhere is this more true than with counseling, which needs to be conducted with an open mind and good listening. Open-ended questions are usually best in eliciting personal narratives. For example, instead of "Are you certain that you want a vasectomy?" "What are your thoughts about having a vasectomy?" "What pressures do you feel to have a vasectomy?" instead of, "Is anyone pressuring you to have a vasectomy?" Yes/No responses limit disclosure whereas unrestricted responses encourage it. Unusual things have been discovered such as the spouse's entire family urging the individual to have a vasectomy.

There are other issues that need to be addressed during counseling. Jeanne Haws, Phyllis Butta and Sally Girvin—A Comprehensive And Efficient Process For Counseling Patients Desiring Sterilization—published in The

Nurse Practitioner in 1997, identified elements unique to sterilization counseling. First and foremost, emphasizing that sterilization is permanent, and is difficult to reverse. Not infrequently, the person has been advised that reversals are very successful. Reversal surgery is expensive and usually not covered by any insurance plan, is not readily available, frequently does not work at least in regards to achieving pregnancy, and can fail after a while due to scarring over. Desire to store sperm is a clear indication that the person is not completely comfortable with the concept of permanent sterilization and must strongly reconsider it. Jeanne Haws and colleagues suggest screening for regret factors, which for males include marital instability, young age (less than 31), choice of vasectomy related to pregnancy or financial crisis, and no children or very young children. If any of these regret factors is present time for reflection and additional counseling is warranted.

According to Jeanne Haws, counseling sessions should also include discussions of alternative contraceptive methods and their effectiveness, interest in and readiness for the procedure, an assessment of relationship functioning preferably with the spouse present, and hormone issues. Regarding the latter, many men equate vasectomy with castration and diminished manhood. Explaining that the testosterone secreting cells remain much the same and the testes still release male hormones into the bloodstream can be very reassuring. It is also advised that both short and long-term complications be explained, and although this overlaps with informed consent, excessive coverage is much better than inadequate coverage as a physician will undoubtedly discover during litigation. Despite the low rate of short-lived early complications, vasectomy results in the highest number of malpractice cases filed against urologists, accounting for over 50% of such litigation! Excellent counseling a month prior to vasectomy helps ensure highly motivated (for the right reasons) patients who fully understand what they might be in for. Any signs of potential regret or hesitancy warrant further counseling. The safest policy is—if there is any doubt, there is no doubt.

INFORMED CONSENT:

Assuming that a person is mentally capable of giving consent, rarely an issue with vasectomy counseling, the criteria for informed consent are satisfied when there has been adequate disclosure of information pertaining to the following:

- Nature of the proposed treatments, preferably aided by diagrams.

- The expected benefits.

- The risks and side effects of treatment.

- Alternative courses of action that could reasonably be pursued.

- The likely consequences of not having the treatment.

The gold standard of disclosure is the information that a reasonable person in the patient's specific situation would want to know to make an informed decision.

Risks of the procedure both short-term and long-term must be carefully outlined, and it is highly recommended that a booklet be prepared and distributed clearly explaining what might occur. Long-term effects must include detailed information on Post-Vasectomy Pain Syndrome. Frequently, perhaps even universally, this "side-effect" is downplayed as "rare" or if present "usually not that much of a problem "and "treatable." Patients must be clearly advised of the potential severity of the condition plus difficulty and enormous cost involved in treating PVPS, and that in the worst cases the testicle is removed at which point pain might be felt in the other testicle. I would like to see it enshrined in legislation that any physician who fails to provide full disclosure about PVPS, including the difficulty and cost associated with treating it, be held financially responsible for any corrective surgery that ensues. If external pressure to have a vasectomy is not present, I wonder how many men would go through with it when they are made fully aware that about 1 in 7 develop chronic pain in the testicles and that for about 1 in 10 the pain is severe plus very difficult and expensive to treat?

Informed consent should be obtained by the physician who will be performing the vasectomy as this person is best able to explain the exact procedure and provide medical details. It also holds the physician fully accountable for this component of the process. I suggest that the informed consent discussion take place approximately a month prior to the date of the procedure, and if at all possible on the same day as the counseling session to limit patient inconvenience and provide as comprehensive an information package as is reasonably possible on one visit. The physician must also take an adequate history of the patient's medical and psychiatric state to identify conditions that might be problematic in conjunction with vasectomy. A physical exam of the scrotum should be mandatory to detect conditions such as a varicocoele (similar to a varicose vein), thickening of the spermatic cord, hydrocele (fluid in a cavity), or epididymal cyst, each of which can make the "simple" vasectomy much more technically challenging, thereby both increasing the risk of side-effects and making the interpretation of any pain symptoms much more difficult.

As amazing as it might sound, some physicians and prominent vasectomy clinics provide both "consultations" and actual vasectomy on the same day—the so-called "Combo" procedure! Sounds like a meal deal at a fast food restaurant. This practice optimizes the income of the provider as payment is usually based on the procedure itself, and setting up an earlier session to counsel and provide information for informed consent diminishes revenues. In addition, true counseling is undoubtedly neglected in this streamlined approach further diminishing the time involvement and costs to the provider.

Those who provide this "Combo" package will undoubtedly say that it is more time friendly to the patient, but anyone who is so busy that they cannot schedule one joint counseling and informed consent session a month prior to surgery, is simply far too busy to have sex making the procedure unnecessary in the first place. Vasectomy lasts a lifetime and patients have a right to digest the information from counseling and the informed consent process well before actual surgery. It appears that physicians, many medical governing bodies, and of course medical malpractice lawyers are content to leave vasectomy as a kind of wild-west saga. Unfortunately, those playing the victim in this ongoing action-drama are not fully aware of the part they are playing.

ADDITIONAL VASECTOMY PROBLEMS

Post-Vasectomy Pain Syndrome is clearly the central focus and relatively little space will be devoted to other real and potential complications of vasectomy, of which there seems to be no shortage. For simplicity sake I will divide them into short-term (limited to the first 3 months), antisperm antibody related, and psychological problems. It is very important to note that sperm granuloma is often considered a side effect of vasectomy, but as we have seen, it is a virtually inevitable outcome of both closed-ended and open-ended vasectomy. To classify an inevitable byproduct of vasectomy as a complication simply reflects inadequate comprehension of the dynamics involved.

SHORT-TERM COMPLICATIONS:

The complications immediately following vasectomy have been quite well studied and a general theme throughout the literature is that vasectomy is "safe." A potential complication of any surgical procedure is wound infection, which sometimes will result in an abscess. Of the studies reviewed there is quite a range with less than 1% reported by William Moss—A Comparison Of Open-Ended Versus Closed-Ended Vasectomies: A Report On 6220 Cases—where patients were just instructed to return or call if any problems arose, a format that could easily have minimized reporting as some patients undoubtedly went to their family doctor or treated the problem on their own.

On the higher end of the range, Manikandan and colleagues—Early And Late Morbidity After Vasectomy: A Comparison Of Chronic Scrotal Pain At 1 And 10 Years—

reported 13% with wound infections requiring antibiotics. Of interest, these researchers did not find any relationship between wound infections and the later development of chronic pain. Their results were based on patients filling out a clearly worded questionnaire that would have produced a much ·more accurate rate than the format used by Moss. Averaging the results from the studies reviewed it appears that perhaps 5% is a reasonable figure for wound infections following vasectomy. Regarding other sources of infection, release from the prostate, seminal vesicles or urinary tract can occasionally occur. These infections do not show any obvious signs such as pus and require different antibiotics than those for superficial skin infections.

Bleeding into a relatively confined space within the scrotal area produces a hematoma. Moss reported less than 1% but patients were only to call or return if there was a problem and many hematomas resolve on their own. The highest rate reported was by Choe and Kirkimo— Questionnaire-Based Outcomes Study Of Nononcological Post-Vasectomy Complications—at 12.6% but they included bleeding without actual hematoma formation. Based on an average of results reported in the studies reviewed, a rate of 1% to 3% is a reasonable expectation with most resolving on their own and only some requiring surgical drainage. Similar to a hematoma but filled with fluid other than blood is a hydrocele. Relatively few studies reported on this complication but the range is from less than 1% to 4%.

Most other immediate aftereffects of vasectomy are slightly less common, including wound separation, hair in the incision, and adhesions. From the realm of the horror zone, there have been a few reported cases of gangrene (Fournier's Gangrene) following vasectomy. Lema reported two cases—Fournier's Gangrene Complicating Vasectomy— in the East African Medical Journal in 2003. In one case a government officer was prescribed antibiotics at the time of vasectomy, but 10 days later he was in so much pain that he could not walk or sit up. Gangrene had set into the scrotum, and part of the penis. Fortunately, he was admitted to a private hospital, a rare occurrence for Africans, started on broad-spectrum antibiotics and operated on. Much of the scrotum and some of the outer portion of the penis were removed. Sophisticated reconstructive surgery was used to repair the scrotum. In the second case involving a peasant farmer, only the scrotum was gangrenous but by mistake the surgeon removed both testicles and hence the man's source of male hormones. It is reasonable to anticipate a major lawsuit if this was to have occurred in the United States, but no such luck for an unlucky African peasant farmer.

ANTISPERM ANTIBODY RELATED CONDITIONS:

The humoral or blood-based immune response to sperm consists of antibody formation. Antisperm antibodies are present in 60% to 70% of men 1 year following their vasectomy and have been found to persist in the circulation for several years. The question arises—Do these circulating antibodies damage any organs such as the heart or prostate? A study by Sotolongo—Immunological Effects Of Vasectomy—published in The Journal Of Urology in 1982, suggested that the answer is—Yes! Monkeys were found to have more atherosclerosis (hardening of the arteries) after vasectomy. Does the same occurrence apply to humans? While all mammals demonstrate antisperm antibodies following vasectomy, the impact of these antibodies appears to be specific to the type of species. In response to the threat of an increased risk for cardiovascular disease following vasectomy, a great deal of fear and research effort has been directed to this topic.

The result of this very extensive and expensive research supports the conclusion that antisperm antibodies do not increase the risk of cardiovascular disease. A major study examining cardiovascular risk by Sean Coady and colleagues—Vasectomy, Inflammation, Atherosclerosis And Long-Term Follow-up For Cardiovascular Diseases: No Association In The Atherosclerosis Risk In Communities Study—published in The Journal Of Urology in 2002, compared 1,050 vasectomized men to just under 3,000 non-vasectomized men. The former group had been vasectomized an average of 16 years earlier, with 20% having it done 20 or more years ago. The rate of diagnosed coronary artery disease and stroke, plus measurements of artery hardening were applied. There was no difference in any of the cardiovascular risk factors between the vasectomized and nonvasectomized groups, and longer duration since vasectomy (20 or more years) did not increase the risk.

Increased risk of prostate cancer has been examined in numerous studies, due to concerns that antisperm antibodies or other mechanisms might damage the prostate following vasectomy. The results of these studies, a review of which could easily fill a book of this length, provides a somewhat confusing picture and one that is certainly less clear than for heart and blood vessel disease. However, it appears reasonable to summarize the results by stating that there is likely no increased risk, other than perhaps for those men with a strong family history of prostate cancer. For example, your father and his father developed it. An increased risk of testicular cancer has also been suggested, but a study involving 73,000 men found no increased risk.

I find it amazing that such a massive research effort has been put into detecting what would likely be a slight increase in risk for diseases that tend to arise later in life, such as cardiovascular disease and prostate cancer, while Post-Vasectomy Pain Syndrome is completely neglected in comparison. Here we have a condition that involves lifelong pain, frequently diminishes the quality of life by making many activities such as sex and sports unpleasant, and affects at least 1 in 7 vasectomized men! Misguided, certainly characterizes this gross error in research direction.

PSYCHOLOGICAL PROBLEMS:

Despite limitations to several studies, there are some clear patterns that emerge regarding the psychology of vasectomy. Foremost is that regret after a vasectomy is predictable when the following apply:

– No children or fewer children than desired.

– Later wishing for more children. Frequently, this occurs when a man has a vasectomy earlier in life, divorces, and then remarries a partner still in her reproductive years. Given the high divorce rate and the low average length of marriage, vasectomy in the twenties or early thirties is easy to regret later on.

– Age less than 30 for what would seem to be obvious reasons.

– Marital difficulties, unstable relationship, and lack of communication. Much as children are no solution to marital problems, vasectomy cannot resolve these problems and might actually worsen them if the man feels pressured by his partner.

– Pressure to have a vasectomy. Some of the studies reviewed make it seem like the decision takes place in an ideal world with both husband and wife sharing the decision 50/50. While this might occur in some cases the reality is often not so ideal. Covert psychological pressures are not uncommon and many men feel guilty if they refuse to have a vasectomy after all their wife went through. There are also overt pressures frequently missed by physicians obtaining consent. Merlin Johnson— Social And Psychological Effects Of Vasectomy— published in The American Journal Of Psychiatry in 1964, reported on 83 men admitted to Seattle Veterans Administration Hospital who received a vasectomy some time prior to admission. In 30 instances the wife, her

74

family, or her physician vigorously pushed for the vasectomy, viewing it as a problem for the husband to solve. In one case the wife's family actually held conferences of sorts essentially making the decision for the husband. Now if that is not marrying into the wrong in-laws I don't know what is. 11 of these men were hospitalized for a psychiatric illness within one year of the vasectomy. Merlin Johnson makes a couple of interesting points— That failure to resolve unwanted pregnancy concerns short of surgical methods, likely reflects problems in the marriage that have passed unnoticed, and that the issue of stress associated with one person undergoing a surgical procedure for the benefit of the other has been largely ignore and needs to be explored.

– Recent experience of a personal crisis. A good rule of thumb is, avoid making a major decision until after a personal crisis is well passed and life is stable. Decisions made during a crisis period are usually poorly informed.

– Practice of religion that does not permit vasectomy.

– The belief that vasectomy = castration. Vasectomy does not seem to interfere with the production and release of male hormones, and hence does not reduce masculinity. However, many men and particularly those of certain cultures, such as Latinos, equate the ability to inseminate females with masculinity. This is not an either or belief and there are varying degrees of adherence to it, something missed in every study reviewed. In other words the belief—Vasectomy makes me less of a man, needs to be evaluated on a scale such as:

1		2	3	4	5	6	7

Not at all true   100% true

I suggest that all vasectomy counselors use this scale and not recommend vasectomy to anyone in the 6 to 7 range. Attitudes can change but typically not from 6-7 to 1-2. Those in the 3 to 5 range will likely respond well to education.

– High interest in sperm banking prior to vasectomy. Interest in this strategy clearly indicates that the man is uncertain about vasectomy, and he should be encouraged not to proceed with it.

I strongly recommend that when even one of these factors is present vasectomy not be performed. Furthermore, it is the responsibility of contraception counselors and physicians performing vasectomy to adequately assess these considerations with each patient.

A relatively unexplored area has to do with the impact of vasectomy on depression and anxiety. Luo Lin and colleagues—Psychological Long-Term Effects Of Sterilization On Anxiety And Depression—published in Contraception in 1996, compared 500 vasectomized men to 500 similar but non-vasectomized men in two counties and two cities in China. They used the Center for Epidemiologic Studies Depression Scale (CES-D Scale) and the Self-Rating Anxiety Scale (SAS). Scores on the depression scale revealed that sterilized men were 4 times as likely to be depressed as were non-sterilized men, particularly higher educated, wealthier, relatively older men who lived in cities. Men fitting this profile also tended to be over 4 times as likely to suffer from anxiety than were men in the non-vasectomized group. They conclude that vasectomy is a risk factor for depression and anxiety and advise that patients be counseled before, during, and after sterilization. The recommendation to counsel after vasectomy is a very interesting one as it might go a long way to prevent or minimize depression and anxiety.

When chronic pain results from vasectomy adverse psychological states can be expected. Schover—Psychological Factors In Men With Genital Pain—published in the Cleveland Clinical Journal Of Medicine in 1990, found that men suffering from testicular pain showed signs of Major Depression (a severe form of depression) and frequently abused chemical substances. Chronic pain patients commonly abuse narcotic medications and other substances as a way of self-medicating for the pain, and also the depressed and anxious mood states that almost invariably arise from ongoing pain conditions. The skeptical response of some physicians to their complaints does not help them cope with the pain and usually worsens symptoms of psychological suffering. Any physician who doubts the suffering of patients with PVPS should volunteer to have sandpaper surgically placed adjacent to the vas, epididymis and testicle on at least one side.

Several studies report little impact of vasectomy on psychological and sexual states and seem to fall in line with the "safe and simple" rhetoric. In an interesting article—A Methodological Critique Of Research On Psychological Effects Of Vasectomy—published in Psychosomatic Medicine in 1974, William Wiest and Lois Janke argue that study design flaws result in a positive bias, or in other words, the studies over-represent the favorable side of vasectomy. One key issue is that most studies rely on questionnaire responses that likely underreport pain and negative results. Men who are suffering might not be as likely to fill out the questionnaire due to preoccupation with their symptoms, or resentment resulting in a lack of desire to cooperate. It would seem at first consideration that men who are suffering should be more interested in responding, but ironically it often goes the other way as they attempt to cope by blocking off reminders of the suffering. Face to face verbal interviews not surprisingly produce higher rates of negative symptom reporting.

William Wiest and Lois Janke also suggest that the high reported satisfaction rate might reflect some trait of men who choose vasectomy—they are "yea-sayers" or otherwise disposed to please the investigator by providing answers they believe are wanted. An important psychological process that also likely plays a role is cognitive dissonance reduction. Cognitive dissonance is a state of psychological tension that arises when two cognitions (thoughts) are incompatible, such as "I want to remain healthy and fit." and "I had a vasectomy that might impair my health and cause suffering." How the mind resolves this unpleasant mental state is by altering one or both of the cognitions so that they align. In this instance a man is unlikely to believe he does not want to remain healthy and fit, nor is he able to deny that a vasectomy occurred. The only way to resolve the dissonance is to downplay any adverse affects by minimizing them to the self and others. This results in a positive response bias with underreporting of negative results. For all these reasons most studies based on questionnaire responses, which are the definite majority, probably underreport psychological and even physical symptoms.

A FAREWELL TO VASECTOMY

How much of a problem is Post-Vasectomy Pain Syndrome? No one is exactly certain since relatively little research has examined this important question. That it is a syndrome producing lifelong pain is no longer possible to dispute. However, the magnitude of the problem is somewhat obscure. Informed estimates place the number of vasectomies worldwide at from 42 to 60 million married couples in 2000 and 100 million men in total as of 2001. Given that the year is now 2006, it is fair to assume well over 100 million vasectomized men. Supporting this figure is the percent of couples in various countries relying on vasectomy. In the United States 11%, Canada 13%, United Kingdom 14%, China 8%, India 7%, Australia 10% and New Zealand a staggering 23%! Considering that between China and India alone there are about 2 billion people, there might well be over 100 million vasectomized men in these two countries alone.

Next we consider the percent of vasectomized men who end up with PVPS. Estimates range from 5% to over 50% but a reasonable figure is 1/7 or about 15% of vasectomized men suffering from PVPS, with perhaps 5% experiencing severe pain. Left untreated the symptoms rarely improve, and certainly not in the more severe range of pain. Treatment is feasible but has limited long-lasting success, and due to availability-cost issues might only be an option for a small percentage of those suffering. Basing our calculation on the conservative figures of 100 million men vasectomized worldwide and 15% with PVPS, 5% with severe pain, 15 million men experience PVPS and 5 million severe lifelong pain symptoms! These numbers are staggering and very difficult to dispute given the conservative figures they are based on.

So why is this not a major issue in medicine in general and urology in particular? An extremely good question to be sure. There is that party line, vasectomy as a "safe and simple procedure." In every area of medicine accepted doctrine has as much to do with politics as it does with the truth and nothing but the truth. When heads of academic departments hold to a certain viewpoint it tends to be the accepted doctrine. Students at all levels are taught that this is the way it is and pass the perspective onto others, editors of academic journals (who are also those running academic departments) decide which articles are published and perhaps not surprisingly favor those consistent with their own viewpoint, and promotions within academic departments are preferentially handed out to those with perspectives in line with the prevailing doctrine.

Vasectomy as a "safe and simple procedure" is the accepted doctrine within most, if not all, academic urology departments. In reviewing the literature, I noted that this very line appeared many times even when the content of the article suggests that vasectomy is not a safe procedure. It almost seems the authors believed the inclusion of this line was necessary for the article to be accepted for publication. If there is one outstanding value to higher education it unquestionably must be to question. Perhaps the world isn't flat, maybe the earth goes around the sun, could ulcers actually be due to bacteria and not stress? To question in a logical fashion is to advance knowledge and science. To accept the generally accepted doctrine is to advance politically.

But why is vasectomy as a "safe and simple procedure" the accepted doctrine within urology? Reports of chronic pain really only started to surface in the 1970's giving the "safe and simple procedure" doctrine a long period to develop unchallenged, and once established in academic departments the accepted doctrine tends to persist. The "safe and simple procedure" doctrine is appealing to most urologists, other surgeons and family physicians who perform vasectomy, because for all our faults we physicians like to believe that we are offering patients a valuable service and now with the larger media sold on the "safe and simple procedure" doctrine, many patients request a vasectomy.

Then there is that source of so many motivations— money. A tremendous amount of money is to be made by performing vasectomies, because while the "safe" part of the accepted doctrine is false, the "simple" is basically accurate. Nancy Hendrix, Sunseet Chauhan and John Morrison— Sterilization And Its Consequences—published in the Obstetrical And Gynecological Survey in 1999, report on costs within the United States. They indicate that at their hospital the cost of vasectomy is $739 and compare it to 1983 US wide figures of $353 to $756. For a procedure that takes a matter of minutes, not a bad return. A standard figure quoted is 500,000 vasectomies in the US per year, at $739 per cut $369 million goes to physicians and clinics per year for providing vasectomies! In addition, there is the income from managing complications and providing routine follow-up assessment. It is no wonder that the party line is not questioned too strongly.

When we look at income to physicians and clinics va-sectomy reversal operations cannot be ignored. Approxi-mately 5% of men consider having their vasectomy reversed with 1% actually doing so and the percent is increasing. Nancy Hendrix and colleagues report that the cost of revers-ing a vasectomy is $9,606 with $2,500 for the actual reversal component. Take 500,000 vasectomies per year and 1% reversal rate, we have $48 million with $12.5 million going directly to surgeons performing the delicate microsurgery, based on values that are currently seven years out of date. Given the demand from patients largely to restore fertility and financial compensation to the service provider, many urologists and general surgeons are getting into the vasectomy reversal business.

Provision of a procedure that is necessary due to another elective (non-urgent) procedure offered by the same surgeon is highly questionable. Particularly so when we consider counseling and informed consent relevant to chronic pain syndromes. At an unconscious level, at least, there is a motivation for surgeons providing vasectomy reversals to minimize the occurrence rate and possible symptoms of Post-Vasectomy Pain Syndrome to prospective vasectomy patients, given the effort required to learn and maintain the vasectomy reversal skills plus the financial compensation for providing it. Due to this conflict of interest I believe that surgeons providing vasectomy reversal should no longer be permitted to provide vasectomies. Observance of the highest standards of counseling and informed consent require no less than this.

In preparing this book I have tried to be objective and limit emotional appeals. However, one issue that needs to be put out there in the strongest of terms is—Many men in less advantaged areas of the world, such as Africa, have little chance of receiving even basic treatment for PVPS, and sophisticated microsurgical reversal or nerve denervation surgery is as likely for them as is training for a space mission. Perhaps removal of one or both testicles requiring relatively little surgical expertise is available, but what a personal price to pay. For the most part men in highly limited financial circumstances, including those in the developed world, will do what the disadvantage usually do—suffer.

Undoubtedly, the comment will be made that men in third world countries, and men in general for that matter, must do their part to limit population expansion. However, a more pressing concern is limiting the spread of HIV and the many other forms of sexually transmitted disease, something that vasectomy does nothing positive for, and might even accelerate by giving some men and women a false sense of security. Personally, I would rather see a few more children born into the world than a child infected with HIV or orphaned when his or her parents succumb to this disease. For those in exclusive and solid relationships, there are always alternatives to cutting, and resorting to cutting might very well reflect difficulties with communication and problem solving within the relationship. Another way of looking at this issue, is that couples successful at finding non-surgical solutions to their pregnancy concern will probably have the communication and problems solving skills required to stay together as a couple.

Do I really expect vasectomy to die off? Yes I do, and I would not be surprised if future generations view it as a crude and barbaric solution to a problem that even today has several alternative solutions. Given the accepted doctrine of vasectomy as a "safe and simple procedure" and the vast sums of money to be made by physicians and clinics providing it, I certainly do not expect a peaceful farewell. However, recognition of Post-Vasectomy Pain Syndrome as the exposed tip of a large and lethal iceberg will help start the ball rolling. When the costs of medical litigation exceed income derived from performing the procedure, major change will undoubtedly ensue. In the meantime, I strongly encourage all who read this to take the "ectomy" out of vas and not wish the cruelest cut of all on anyone.

BIBLIOGRAPHY

Ahmed, I., Rasheed, S., White, C. & Shaikh, N. (1997). The Incidence Of Post-Vasectomy Chronic Testicular Pain And The Role Of Nerve Stripping (Denervation) Of The Spermatic Cord In Its Management. British Journal Of Urology, 79, 269-270.

Alexander, N. & Schmidt, S. (1977). Incidence Of Antisperm Antibody Levels And Granulomas In Men. Fertility And Sterility, 28(6), 655-657.

Amundsen, G. & Ramakrishnan, K. (2004). Vasectomy: A "Seminal" Analysis. Southern Medical Journal, 97(1), 54-60.

Babayan, R. & Krane, R. (1986). Vasectomy: What Are Community Standards? Sterility & Fertility, 27(4), 328-330.

Belker, A. (1987). Vasectomy Reversal. Urologic Clinics Of North America, 14(1), 155-166.

Chen, T. & Ball, R. (1991). Epididymectomy For Post-Vasectomy Pain: Histological Review. British Journal Of Urology, 68, 407-413.

Choe, J. & Kirkemo, A. (1996). Questionnaire-Based Outcomes Study Of Nononcological Post-Vasectomy Complications. The Journal Of Urology, 155, 1284-1286.

Christiansen, C. & Sandlow, J. (2003). Testicular Pain Following Vasectomy: A Review Of Postvasectomy Pain Syndrome. Journal Of Andrology, 24(3), 293-298.

Clenney, T. & Higgins, J. (1999). Vasectomy Techniques. American Family Physician, 60(1), 137-146.

Coady, S., Sharrett, A., Zheng, Z., Evans, G. & Heiss, G. (2002). Vasectomy, Inflammation, Atherosclerosis And Long-Term Follow-Up For Cardiovascular Diseases: No Associations In The Atherosclerosis Risk In Communities Study. The Journal Of Urology, 167, 204-207.

Dias, P. (1983). The Long-Term Effects Of Vasectomy On Sexual Behavior. Acta Psychiatric Scandanavia, 67, 333-338.

Doiron, K, Legare, C., Fabrice, S. & Sullivan, R. (2002). Effect Of Vasectomy On Gene Expression In The Epididymis Of Cynomolgus Monkey. Biology Of Reproduction, 68, 781-788.

Errey, B. & Edwards, I. (1986). Open-Ended Vasectomy: An Assessment. Fertility And Sterility, 45(6), 843-846.

Esho, J., Cass, A. & Ireland, G. (1973). Morbidity Associated With Vasectomy. The Journal Of Urology, 110, 413-415.

Flickinger, C. (1985). The Effects Of Vasectomy On The Testis. The New England Journal Of Medicine, 313(20), 1283-1284.

Gingell, C., Crosby, D. & Carroll, R. (2001). Review Of The Complications And Medicolegal Implications Of Vasectomy. Postgraduate Medical Jornal, 77, 656-659.

Giovannucci, E. (2001). Medical History And Etiology Of Prostate Cancer. Epidemiologic Reviews, 23(1), 159-166.

Granitsiotis, P. & Kirk, D. (2004). Chronic Testicular Pain: An Overview. European Urology, 45, 430-436.

Guillebaud, P. & Budd, D. (1984). Complications Of Vasectomy: Review Of 16,000 Patients. British Journal Of Urology, 56, 745-748.

Haws, J., Butta, P. & Girvin, S. (1997). A Comprehensive And Efficient Process For Counseling Patients Desiring Sterilization. The Nurse Practitioner, 22(6), 52-66.

Hendrix, N., Chauhan, S. & Morrison, J. (1999). Sterilization And Its Consequences. Obstetrical And Gynecological Survey, 54(12), 766-777.

Jarow, J., Budin, R., Dym, M., Zirkin, B., Noren, S. & Marshall, F. (1985), Quantitative Pathologic Changes In The Human Testis After Vasectomy. The New England Journal Of Medicine, 313(20), 1252-1256.

Jarvis, L. & Dubbins, P. (1989). Changes In The Epididymis After Vasectomy: Sonographic Findings. American Journal Of Roentgen., 152, 531-534.

Johnson, M. (1964). Social And Psychological Effects Of Vasectomy. The American Journal Of Psychiatry, November, 482-486.

Kwart, A. & Coffey, D. (1973). Sperm Granulomas: An Adverse Effect Of Vasectomy. The Journal Of Urology, 110, 416-422.

Labrecque, M., Nazerali, H., Mondor, M., Fortin, V. & Nasution, M. (2002). Effectiveness And Complications Associated With 2 Vasectomy Occlusion Techniques. The Journal Of Urology, 168, 2495-2498.

Leader, A., Axelrad, S., Frankowski, R. & Mumford, S. (1974). Complications Of 2,711 Vasectomies. The Journal Of Urology, 111, 365-369.

Lema, V. (2003). Fournier's Gangrene Complicating Vasectomy. East African Medical Journal, 80(9), 492-496.

Levine, L. & Matkov, T. (2001). Microsurgical Denervation Of The Spermatic Cord As Primary Surgical Treatment Of Chronic Orchialgia. Journal Of Urology, 165, 1927-1929

Lin, L., Shi-Zhong, W., Changmin, Z., Qifu, F., Kegiang, L. & Goliang, S. (1996). Psychological Long-Term Effects Of Sterilization On Anxiety And Depression. Contraception, 54, 345-357.

McCormack, M. & Lapointe, S. (1988). Physiological Consequences And Complications Of Vasectomy. Canadian Medical Association Journal, 138, 223-225.

McDonald, S. (2000). Cellular Responses To Vasectomy. International Review Of Cytology, 199, 295-339.

McMahon, A., Buckley, J., Talylor, A., Lloyd, S., Deane, R. & Kirk, D. (1992). Chronic Testicular Pain Following Vasectomy. British Journal Of Urology, 69, 188-191.

Manikandan, R., Srirangam, S., Pearson, E. & Collins, G. (2004). Early And Late Morbidity After Vasectomy: A Comparison Of Chronic Scrotal Pain At 1 And 10 Years. BJU International, 93, 571-574.

Meng, M., Black, L., Cha, I., Ljung, B, Pera, R. & Turek, P. (2001). Impaired Spermatogenesis In Men With Congenital Absence Of The Vas Deferens. Human Reproduction, 16(3), 529-533.

Moss, W. (1992). A Comparison Of Open-End Versus Closed-End Vasectomies: A Report On 6220 Cases. Contraception, 46, 521-525.

Myers, S., Mershon, C. & Fuchs, E. (1997). Vasectomy Reversal For The Treatment Of The Post-Vasectomy Pain Syndrome. The Journal Of Urology, 157, 518-520.

Nagler, H. & Rotman, M. (2002). Predictive Parameters For Microsurgical Reconstruction. Urologic Clinics Of North America, 29, 913-919.

Nangia, A., Myles, J. & Thomas, A. (2000). Vasectomy Reversal For The Post-Vasectomy Pain Syndrome: A Clinical And Histological Evaluation. The Journal Of Urology, 164, 1939-1942.

Nash, J. & Rich, J. (1972). The Sexual Aftereffects Of Vasectomy. Fertility And Sterility, 23(10), 715-718.

Nistal, M., Riestra, M., Galmes-Belmonte, I. & Paniagua, R. (1999). Testicular Biopsy In Patients With Obstructive Azoospermia. The American Journal Of Surgical Pathology, 23(12), 1546-1554.

O'Conor, V. (1948). Anastomosis Of Vas Deferens After Purposeful Division For Sterility. Journal Of The American Medical Association, 136-62.

Pabst, R., Martin, O. & Lippert, H. (1979). Is The Low Fertility Rate After Vasovasostomy Caused By Nerve Resection During Vasectomy? Fertility And Sterility, 31(3), 316-320.

Padmore, D., Norman, R. & Millard, O. (1996). Analyses Of Indications For And Outcomes Of Epididymectomy. Journal Of Urology, 156(1), 95-96.

Pardanani, D., Nivrutti, G. & Pawar, H. (1976). Some Gross Observations Of The Epididymides Following Vasectomy: A Clinical Study. Fertility And Sterility, 27(3), 267-270.

Pryor, J. & Howards, S. (1987). Varicocele. Urologic Clinics Of North America, 14(3), 499-513.

Sandlow, J., Westefeld, J., Maples, M. & Scheel, K. (2001). Psychological Correlates Of Vasectomy. Fertility And Sterility, 75(3), 544-548.

Schachter, D., Kleinman, I. & Harvey, W. (2005). Informed Consent And Adolescents. The Canadian Journal Of Psychiatry, 50(9), 534-540.

Schmidt, S. (1979). Spermatic Granuloma: An Often Painful Lesion. Fertility And Sterility, 31(2), 178-181.

Schmidt, S. & Brueschke, E. (1976). Anatomical Sizes Of The Human Vas Deferens After Vasectomy. Fertility And Sterility, 27(3), 271-274.

Schover, L. (1990). Psychological Factors In Men With Genital Pain. Cleveland Clinical Journal Of Medicine, 57(8), 697-700.

Schroeder-Printzen, I., Diemer, T. & Weidner, W. (2003). Vasovasostomy. Urologia Internationalis, 70, 101-107.

Schwingl, P. & Guess, H. (2000). Safety And Effectiveness Of Vasectomy. Fertility And Sterility, 73(5), 923-936.

Selikowitz, S. & Schned, A. (1985). A Late Post-Vasectomy Syndrome. The Journal Of Urology, 134, 494-497.

Shafik, A. (1996). Electrovasogram In Normal And Vasectomized Men And Patients With Obstructive Azoospermia And Absent Vas Deferens. Archives Of Andrology, 36, 67-79.

Shandling, B. & Janik, J. (1981). The Vulnerability Of The Vas Deferens. Journal Of Pediatric Surgery, 16(4), 461-464.

Shapiro, E. & Silber, S. (1979). Open-Ended Vasectomy, Sperm Granuloma, And Postvasectomy Orchialgia. Fertility And Sterility, 32(5), 546-550.

Shiraishi, K., Naito, K. & Yoshida, K. (2001). Vasectomy Impairs Spermatogenesis Through Germ Cell Apoptosis Mediated By The p53-Bax Pathway In Rats. The Journal Of Urology, 166, 1565-1571.

Shiraishi, K., Takihara, H. & Naito, K. (2002). Influence Of Interstitial Fibrosis On Spermatogenesis After Vasectomy And Vasovasotomy. Contraception, 65, 245-249.

Silber, S. (1977). Microscopic Vasectomy Reversal. Fertility And Sterility, 28(11), 1191-1202.

Silber, S. (1978). Vasectomy And Vasectomy Reversal. Fertility And Sterility, 29(2), 125-140.

Silber, S. (1979). Epididymal Extravasation Following Vasectomy As A Cause For Failure Of Vasectomy Reversal. Fertility And Sterility, 31(3), 309-315.

Silber, S. (1981). Reversal Of Vasectomy And The Treatment Of Male Infertility. Urologic Clinics Of North America, 8, 53-62.

Sneyd, M., Cox, B., Paul, C. & Skegg, D. (2001). High Prevalence Of Vasectomy In New Zealand. Contraception, 64, 155-159.

Soderdahl, D. (1982). Vasectomy: "The Most Unkindest Cut Of All"? Surgery, Gynecology & Obstetrics, 155, 734-736.

Sotolongo, J. (1982). Immunocological Effects Of Vasectomy. Journal Of Urology, 127(6), 1063-1066.

Starling, J., Harms, B., Schroeder, M. & Eichman, P. (1987). Diagnosis And Treatment Of Genitofemoral And Ilioinguinal Entrapment Neuralgia. Surgery, 102(4), 581-586.

Thomas, A. (1987). Vasoepididymostomy. Urologic Clinics Of North America, 14(3), 527-538.

Trussell, J., Guilbert, E. & Hedley, A. (2003). Sterilization Failure, Sterilization Reversal, And Pregnancy After Sterilization Reversal In Quebec. Obstetrics & Gynecology, 101(4), 677-684.

Weiske, W. (2001). Vasectomy. Andrologia, 33, 125-134.

West, A., Leung, H. & Powell, P. (2000). Epididymectomy Is An Effective Treatment For Scrotal Pain After Vasectomy. BJU International, 85(9), 1097-1099.

Whyte, J., Sarrat, R., Cisneros, A., Whyte, A., Mazo, R., Torres, A. & Lazaro, J. (2000). The Vasectomized Testis. International Surgery, 85, 167-174.

Wiest, W. & Janke, L. (1974). A Methodological Critique Of Research On Psychological Effects Of Vasectomy. Psychosomatic Medicine, 36(5), 438-449.

Yarbro, E. & Howards, S. (1987). Vasovasostomy. Urologic Clinics Of North America, 14(3), 515-526.

INDEX

epididymitis, 15-17, 32-36
extravasation (of sperm) 12-20, 25
hydrostatic pressure (backpressure), 8-9, 14-18, 23, 25-26, 37
inflammation, 15-17, 40-41
sperm granuloma, 11, 14-20, 25-26, 29-30, 38-39, 46, 52-53, 57-58

Epididymectomy, 14-17, 59-60

Errey, B., 46-47

Fertility (reproduction), 21-22, 52-54

Fibrous Tissue (Fibrosis),
adhesions, 58
interstitial (connective) tissue, 17, 20-24, 56-57
nerve entrapment, 17-18, 38-43, 57-59
nerve irritation/inflammation, 11-12, 17-18, 20, 39-41, 48, 57-60

Haws, J., 65-66

Hematoma, 48, 71

Hendrix, N., 81-82

Hydrostatic Pressure (backpressure),
vas, 9-14, 37, 45-46
epididymis, 8-9, 14-18, 23, 25-26, 37
efferent tubules, 19, 25-26, 37
testicles, 1, 10, 20-26, 36-37, 40-41, 47

Immune system (immunological effects),
Atherosclerosis, 12, 72-73
cell-based response, 11-13, 18-19, 47-48
humoral (blood borne response), 11-13, 17-22, 37, 47-48, 72-73

secretions, 6-8, 34
vasectomy, 8, 10, 44-45, 51

Questionnaire (Surveys), 30-35, 77-78
positive response bias, 77-78

Schmidt, S., 11-12, 29, 38-39, 45, 52-53

Schover, L., 77

Selikowitz, S., 15-17, 36-38, 60-61

Seminal Vesicles, 7, 71

Sertoli Cells, 4, 20-26

Shafik, A., 13-14, 37

Shandling, B., 10, 40-41

Shapiro, E., 15, 19, 29-30, 36, 38, 48

Shiraishi, K., 22-23

Silber, S., 9, 11, 15, 18-19, 24, 29-30, 36, 38-39, 43, 45

Sotolongo, J., 72

Sperm (spermatozoa),
banking, 76
count, 4-5
extravasation, 1, 11-13, 16-18, 25-26, 38-39, 42-43, 60-61
motility, 5-7, 19-26, 45-46, 53-59
Sertoli cells, 4, 23-26

Sperm Granuloma,
asymptomatic, 11-12, 36, 45-47
cystic, 15-16
of epididymis, 11, 14-20, 25-26, 29-30, 38-39, 46, 52-53, 57-58

of vas, 11, 18-19, 29-30, 38-39, 47-48
recanalization, 44-49
symptomatic, 12, 29-30, 32-33, 38-43, 47-49, 52-53

Starling, J., 43, 59

Testicle,
hydrostatic pressure (backpressure), 1, 10, 20-26, 36-37, 40-41, 47
Leydig cells, 4, 24, 66
removal of (orchiectomy), 1, 50, 61-62, 71-72
seminiferous tubules, 4, 20-23
Sertoli cells, 4, 20-26

Testosterone, 4, 24-25, 61-62

Thomas, A., 55-56

Varicocele, 68

Vas Deferens (Vas),
action potentials (AP), 13-14, 37
ductules (Vasitis Nodosum), 45-46
electrovasogram, 13-14
hydrostatic pressure (backpressure), 9-14, 37, 45-46
lumen, 6-7, 10-11, 13, 45-46
muscles layers, 6-7, 10-11, 13, 18, 38-39, 52
pacesetter potentials (PP), 13-14
sperm granuloma, 11, 18-19, 29-30, 38-39, 47-48
vasoarrhythmia, 13-14

Vasectomy (Vasectomized),
anxiety, 76-77
castration (fear), 61-62, 75
cautery, 8, 44-45
clipping, 8
closed-ended, 8, 11-12, 18, 24-25, 37, 44-49, 57
"combo" procedure, 68-69
complications (early), 3, 11-12, 44-49, 66, 70-72